Praise for *The Women's Fibromyalgia Toolkit*

". . . a practical toolkit for managing fibromyalgia that distills the wealth of current recommendations into a manageable individualized program. It will be useful to all fibromyalgia patients who feel overwhelmed by the barrage of recommendations that emanate from their friends and the media and the press."

Robert M. Bennett, MD, Professor of Medicine and Nursing,
Oregon Health & Science University, Portland, OR

". . . Finally we have a book that tells us that fibro is a real biological condition. I don't know about you, but those words are music to my ears! I've been to many health care professionals over the years who have said that I need to 'learn to live with it.' Whatever 'it' is! Well, this book gives lots of techniques so that we can take charge of our lives and tell fibro that we are in the driver's seat! And you know what? That gives me lots of hope that today I will be able to feel better than I did yesterday and tomorrow will be even better. . . ."

Patricia Tirrell, CRA, CPDT-KA,
Tellington TTouch Companion Animal Practitioner

"From pre-diagnosis to support groups, how to talk with your doctor or what supplements might be useful, this book provides you with the tools to be an active participant in your own health care. As a medical professional I found the content to be current, well-researched, and documented in a way that was not too difficult for the average person to comprehend. As a patient diagnosed with fibromyalgia for more than 20 years, I found the information to be both practical and sensitive. I am sure that readers will reach for this book time and again to find just the resource or advice to help them live life to the fullest despite fibromyalgia."

Sue Ann Bland, RN

". . . provides a solid scientific and clinical outline for understanding the management of this consuming malady. Fibromyalgia is more than just widespread pain, and its effective management requires an educated patient. This book provides that education and allows the patient to look beyond the false promises of quick fixes of promised cures. It highlights the treatments that will improve their function and quality of life."

Michael Duren Ready, MD,
Scott and White Clinic, Temple, TX

"I am absolutely amazed at how much my life will be changed for the better just by reading this book. The readability was outstanding. . . . very informative and thorough, covering everything anyone with this disease should know. I thought fibromyalgia is just a pain disease and that any other symptoms or problems I am having were just in my head. I am so relieved to know that the other problems I am having are part of having fibromyalgia. And now, with the knowledge I have gained from the book I can manage and even conquer these symptoms.

. . . a must-read book for anyone who has fibromyalgia. . . ."

Kerri Stomas

"(I feel) elated that such a useful, down-to-earth, easily understandable, and balanced resource exists for my patients and the many thousands of patients, families, and health care practitioners who struggle with this common condition. They have truly listened to their patients, know the research on fibromyalgia and its treatment, have had their own deep practical experience with it, and have an earnest interest in empowering patients . . . teaches the reader what we know about the disease process, its physical and emotional impact, and the journey of diagnosis and treatment; practical physical therapy and exercise approaches, complete with photographs; the issue of sleep; how to cope during pregnancy; medications, diet, and supplements; and practical aspects of putting a self-management plan in place. . . ."

Philip Mease MD, Director, Rheumatology Research,
Swedish Medical Center; Clinical Professor,
University of Washington School of Medicine, Seattle, OR

"A fibromyalgia diagnosis doesn't have to be a bewildering journey through chronic pain, medical visits, medicines, and other treatment plans, especially with a helpful resource like *The Woman's Fibromyalgia Toolkit*. This book offers invaluable information for patients and practitioners alike. . . . so the practical summaries and comprehensive tracking logs are great tools for measuring the impact of symptoms, exercise, and relaxation. . . . Drs. Marcus and Deodhar offer hope, understanding, and a useful plan of action for millions who suffer from fibromyalgia—75 to 90 percent of whom are women."

Sheryl Lynn Sochoka,
Marywood Magazine, *Marywood University*

". . . Throughout my 15+ years of working with fellow fibromyalgia patients, my goal has been to educate, encourage, and empower them. This book accomplishes all three.

Education—Who gets fibromyalgia? What causes it? Questions every fibromyalgia patient asks are tackled head on. The multiple symptoms that accompany fibromyalgia are broken down and their biological underpinnings explained in an easy-to-understand format. Then the most effective treatment options available, both traditional and alternative, are discussed indepth. . . .

Encouragement—After reading this book, I felt understood and encouraged. Not only is fibromyalgia validated as a real physical illness with multiple biological abnormalities, but the medical explanations are backed up by solid research that should impress even the most hardened skeptic. Also encouraging is the assurance that fibromyalgia symptoms can be brought under control.

Empowerment—Knowledge is power and this book provides a wealth of knowledge about fibromyalgia. In addition, the tips for communicating effectively with your doctor and the logs for tracking symptoms and treatments are essential tools that empower women to take an active role in managing their fibromyalgia.

. . . a must read for every woman with fibromyalgia. . . ."

Karen Lee Richards, Co-founder,
National Fibromyalgia Association;
Chronic Pain Expert, The HealthCentral Network

The Woman's Fibromyalgia Toolkit

Manage Your Symptoms and Take Control of Your Life

Dawn A. Marcus, MD
Professor
Department of Anesthesiology
University of Pittsburgh
Pittsburgh, Pennsylvania

Atul Deodhar, MD
Professor
Division of Arthritis & Rheumatic Diseases
Oregon Health & Science University
Portland, Oregon

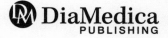

DiaMedica
PUBLISHING

DiaMedica Publishing, 150 East 61st Street, New York, NY 10065

Visit our website at www.diamedicapub.com

ISBN: 978-0-9823219-6-6 (print)
ISBN: 978-1-936832-16-3 (e-book)

Library of Congress Cataloging-in-Publication Data is available from the publisher.

DiaMedica titles are available for bulk purchase, special promotions, and premiums. For more information please contact the publisher through the publisher's website: www.diamedicapub.com.

Disclaimer:
The content in this book is not intended as a substitute for medical or professional counseling and advice. The reader is encouraged to consult his or her physicians and therapists on all health matters, especially symptoms that may require professional diagnosis and/or medical attention.

Book design: TypeWriting
Cover design: Gopa & Ted2
Editors: Jessica Bryan and Joann Woy

Contents

Part II
Fibromyalgia Symptoms and
The Science Behind the Disease

Part III
Fibromyalgia Treatments That Really Work

Part IV
Putting Knowledge Into Practice

Preface

Have you ever been told, "It's only fibromyalgia?" But if you are a woman with fibromyalgia, you know that it's more than "just a pain problem." Although pain is certainly one of the hallmarks of fibromyalgia, this disorder is, in fact, a *syndrome* that includes a wide range of unpleasant and often disabling symptoms that can sap your energy, strength, and focus. Having fibromyalgia can impact your everyday life, your career, relationships with family and friends, and even how you think about yourself.

Fibromyalgia can be especially frustrating because the symptoms are often unpredictable, sometimes flaring up for no particular reason and at inconvenient times. When you're already in pain and feeling fatigued because of fibromyalgia, bouts of bowel or bladder symptoms, migraines, or anxiety can make it difficult to cope. Explaining fibromyalgia to friends, family—and even health care providers—can also be challenging because, in many ways, fibromyalgia is an invisible disability. Although pain, poor sleep, fatigue, and other symptoms may keep you from doing what you'd like or need to do, to the outside world you may look perfectly healthy.

There *is* good news. Doctors are beginning to understand more about the complex symptoms typically experienced by people with fibromyalgia, as well as *why* some women get fibromyalgia. Research clearly proves that fibromyalgia is a very real condition, involving a wide range of biological abnormalities, including changes in nerves, muscles, and the substances involved in inflammation that produce pain and other symptoms. Research also suggests there may be important genetic factors that explain why some people may be more susceptible to developing fibromyalgia. The other good news is that, although there is no cure for fibromyalgia, there *are* effective treatments.

Fibromyalgia has become an area of increased interest both for physicians and medical researchers. Doctors are developing new methods for identifying and understanding fibromyalgia symptoms. At the same time, researchers are carefully evaluating which treatments might be most effective by testing both drug and non-drug therapies in well-designed studies.

We developed *The Woman's Fibromyalgia Toolkit* as a guide to managing the symptoms of fibromyalgia, learning how to identify it, understanding what causes it, and what treatments are worth trying. If you have fibromyalgia, it's important to know that most women need to try a variety of treatments before finding the combination that works best for them.

The Woman's Fibromyalgia Toolkit can help you take control of your fibromyalgia symptoms. You'll learn what to expect from the disease and how to most effectively share your concerns with your health care providers. You'll also find step-by-step instructions for using effective non-drug treatments, including exercises, yoga, and relaxation techniques—which research consistently shows are among the most effective fibromyalgia therapies. You'll also learn which nutritional supplements might be worth a try and what to expect from prescription medications.

Fibromyalgia is a complex condition that probably won't get better by just taking a pill. Effective fibromyalgia treatment usually requires a holistic, comprehensive approach that addresses sleep patterns, exercise habits, and mood, in addition to drug therapies. Tailoring these treatments to symptoms is essential, and although exercise is helpful for most women with fibromyalgia, it's important to develop an exercise program that can be started and advanced without causing undue fibro flares. *The Woman's Fibromyalgia Toolkit* provides a broad sample of tools to help you discover the most effective treatment strategy for *your* fibromyalgia symptoms. You'll also learn what you need to do when you're planning for pregnancy, so you can use safe and effective treatments while trying to get pregnant, during pregnancy, and after the baby's born, when you might be nursing.

You don't have to let fibromyalgia control your life—take charge by learning what causes fibromyalgia, the common symptoms, how to share your concerns with your doctor, and the treatments that are most likely to be helpful. *The Woman's Fibromyalgia Toolkit* offers clear, practical instructions to help you change your life and take back control.

If you have comments, suggestions, or questions about fibromyalgia, please contact Dr. Marcus at www.dawnmarcusmd.com.

Acknowledgments

The authors would like to thank the many patients who have opened their lives to us to help educate us about what it truly means to live with fibromyalgia. We are indebted to Karen Lee Richards for her thoughtful review and the insightful advice she provided to make this book the ideal guide for women with fibromyalgia.

The authors would also like to thank Dawn Buse, PhD, of the Albert Einstein College of Medicine, for providing information and direction for the psychological treatments described in this book; yoga expert and trainer Melissa Watts for providing yoga instructions and expertise; and Cheryl Noethiger for demonstrating the exercise routines.

About the Authors

Dawn Marcus, MD, is a board-certified neurologist and professor at the University of Pittsburgh Medical Center. She specializes in pain management, with a special focus on fibromyalgia research and treatment. Dr. Marcus has been the lead researcher for numerous studies investigating women's issues in pain management and gender differences in the pain experience. Her research has also focused on the holistic treatment of fibromyalgia and other pain complaints, including non-drug, complementary, and alternative treatments.

Atul Deodhar, MD, is a rheumatologist who treats patients with a broad range of rheumatologic and autoimmune disorders, including fibromyalgia. He is Professor of Medicine and the Director of Rheumatology Clinics at Oregon Health & Science University (OHSU). Dr. Deodhar started the first university-based fibromyalgia specialty clinic in 2001 at OHSU for the comprehensive assessment and treatment of fibromyalgia. He has been involved with numerous research studies with fibromyalgia patients, including hormonal changes with the disease and evaluations of both drug and non-drug treatments.

Drs. Marcus and Deodhar are the authors of *Fibromyalgia: A Practical Clinical Guide*, a definitive guide to the treatment of fibromyalgia for health care providers.

Part I

The Basics

About Fibromyalgia

Do you ever feel as if no one really understands your fibromyalgia? Do you feel that your family, friends, co-workers, and even your doctors don't really believe you have problems with pain, fatigue, and sleep disturbance? You should know that you're not alone—fibromyalgia affects 2–3 percent of adults in the United States, Canada, South America, and Europe.

WHAT IS FIBROMYALGIA?

The term *fibromyalgia* comes from the Latin root *fibro-* for fibrous or connective tissue, and the Greek roots *myo-* for muscles and *algos* for pain. So, *fibromyalgia* literally means a pain that affects the muscles and connective tissues. This pain is likely to be widespread, because the body is basically made up of muscles and connective tissue.

Fibromyalgia Is More Than Pain

The name *fibromyalgia* doesn't fully describe the many disabling symptoms that people typically experience with the disease. A survey of people with fibromyalgia found that pain was only part of the disability caused by the syndrome:

FIBROMYALGIA FACT AND FICTION

Fibromyalgia Myths	Fibromyalgia Facts
Fibromyalgia is very rare.	Fibromyalgia affects 2–3 of every 100 adults in the Americas and Europe.
Fibromyalgia only affects women.	Fibromyalgia affects women 3 times more often than men, but men can also be affected.
Fibromyalgia is something only young or middle-aged women complain about.	The average age when women start experiencing the symptoms of fibromyalgia is approximately 45; however, fibromyalgia can persist as women grow older.
Fibromyalgia is just a little pain problem.	Women with fibromyalgia typically have a wide range of troublesome symptoms that can significantly affect their work, family, and enjoyment of life. Fibromyalgia symptoms are often quite disabling.

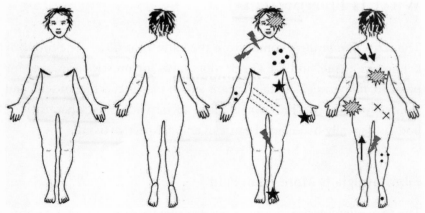

Mark the drawing on the left to show where you often have pain. (This drawing of the human body can be downloaded from www.diamedicapub.com/the-womans -fibromyalgia-toolkit/. You can use different symbols to show different types of pain. The drawing on the right shows how a typical person with fibromyalgia might complete this drawing. Share this drawing with your doctor to help you describe your unique pain pattern.

- ▶ Nine in ten have pain.
- ▶ Nine in ten also have problems with fatigue and stiff joints.
- ▶ Eight in ten experience weakness.
- ▶ Seven in ten have problems with sleep.
- ▶ More than half have headaches.
- ▶ Half also report sore eyes.
- ▶ Four in ten have problems with dizziness.
- ▶ Three in ten have problems with breathlessness.

Mood problems, such as depression or anxiety, are also common, affecting approximately two of three people with fibromyalgia.

Although fibromyalgia is usually referred to as a *chronic pain syndrome*, in some cases, other symptoms may be more of a problem. In one study of fibromyalgia in women, problems with fatigue were more-

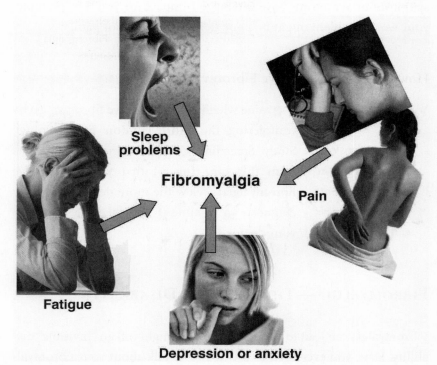

Fibromyalgia typically includes a broad range of unpleasant and often disabling symptoms.

significant than pain because of their effects on quality of life. Another study showed that poor sleep was the worst problem, and that sleep difficulties increased pain and fatigue. This interaction among pain, sleep, and fatigue can result in a vicious spiral of disability.

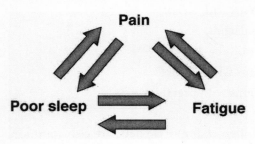

Pain

Poor sleep **Fatigue**

The most common, disabling symptoms of fibromyalgia are pain, poor sleep, and fatigue. Each of these symptoms causes its own problems, and each can aggravate the severity of other common fibromyalgia problems.

Breaking out of the cycle of pain, poor sleep, and fatigue often requires attention to each of these problems. So, be sure to share *all* your troublesome fibromyalgia symptoms with your doctor. Also, be sure to let her know which symptom or symptoms have the biggest impact for you. For example, your worst problem might be poor sleep or fatigue, not pain.

How Do I Know If I Have Fibromyalgia?

You should be able to determine whether you may have fibromyalgia by completing the short London Epidemiology Study Screening Questionnaire. If the results from this quiz suggest that you might have fibromyalgia, review the more detailed tools for diagnosis in Chapter 4 and take the results to your doctor.

Pain, poor sleep, and fatigue are the primary complaints of many people with fibromyalgia.

FIBROMYALGIA—THE INVISIBLE DISABILITY

Fibromyalgia can lead to what some people might call an "invisible" disability. Have you ever been to the doctor to talk about your fibromyalgia symptoms, and after your examination, he said, "But you look

THE LONDON FIBROMYALGIA EPIDEMIOLOGY STUDY SCREENING QUESTIONNAIRE

Answer these questions about your symptoms over the past 3 months.

Pain

Have you had pain in muscles, bones, or joints lasting at least 1 week? ☐ YES ☐ NO

Have you had pain in your shoulders, arms, or hands? On which side? Right, left, or both? ☐ YES ☐ NO

Have you had pain in your legs or feet? On which side? Right, left, or both? ☐ YES ☐ NO

Have you had pain in your neck, chest, or back? ☐ YES ☐ NO

You may have fibromyalgia if you answered "yes" to all four pain questions, and you have pain that affects both the right and left sides of your body.

Fatigue

Do you often feel tired or fatigued? ☐ YES ☐ NO

Does tiredness or fatigue significantly limit your activities? ☐ YES ☐ NO

If you answered "yes" to both fatigue questions, you probably have chronic, debilitating fatigue. This can be part of fibromyalgia.

Adapted from White, et al. *J Rheumatol.* 1999;26:880–4.

terrific!"? When you're able to walk, touch your toes, and move your arms and legs, you may appear to be normal and healthy to the outside world—including your doctors. But looks can be deceiving. Even though most people with fibromyalgia don't have *visible* signs of disability—such as wheelchairs, walkers, and canes—the impact of fibromyalgia is very real.

Most people with fibromyalgia are motivated, hardworking, and often very successful. These people are good patients in terms of follow-

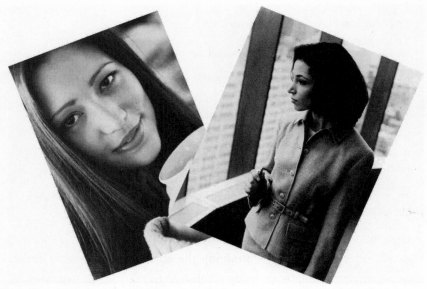

On the outside, people with fibromyalgia often look fine to family, friends, co-workers, and even health care providers. They can often do things such as walk briskly, bend and stretch, and pass the doctor's tests for strength, sensation, and reflexes. They are often able to manage their homes and work by hiding the disabling symptoms they experience every day.

ing through with treatment and consistently working on getting better. Unfortunately, looking good on the outside while feeling terrible on the inside can sometimes cause others—including your doctors—to overlook the significant impact of fibromyalgia on your life.

In an interesting study conducted at the Rehabilitation Foundation Limburg in the Netherlands, scientists compared quality of life in people with fibromyalgia to those with other chronic pain problems. As you might guess, quality of life was substantially lower in the fibromyalgia group compared with healthy people without pain. What was perhaps more surprising was that quality of life was worse with fibromyalgia than with other common painful conditions, such as chronic low back pain and rheumatoid arthritis. The comparison with rheumatoid arthritis was especially interesting because rheumatoid arthritis also causes widespread pain and a range of other symptoms, including stiffness and fatigue. Unlike fibromyalgia, people with rheumatoid arthritis develop joint damage and deformities over time, so they may have a highly visible disability. Despite "looking worse," however, people with rheumatoid arthritis are actually less affected by their symptoms than are those with fibromyalgia.

FIBROMYALGIA IS UNPREDICTABLE

Fibromyalgia symptoms are also unpredictable. Never knowing what you might experience from one day to the next—whether tomorrow will be a good or bad day—adds to the disability of the syndrome. Scientists have been studying the effects of knowing when something bad will occur—or not—by studying the effects of predictable versus unpredictable events. In an study published in the journal *Neuroimage* in 2011, researchers from the Laureate Institute for Brain Research in Tulsa, Oklahoma, tested the responses people had when facing predictable or unpredictable threats.

In their experiment, healthy adults were immersed in virtual reality environments. While investigating each environment, they might receive electric shocks. In one environment, they never got shocked. In another, they only got shocked after they heard a warning tone. In the third, they could be shocked at any time without warning—and yes, people *did* actually sign up for this experiment! As expected, anxiety levels were significantly higher when people knew they were at risk for unpredictable shocks.

Anticipation of unpredictable threats—such as fibro flares—often leads to an increase in sustained anxiety and fear due to activation of specific regions in the brain.

The results of brain scans conducted during the tests were even more interesting. Although the shocks were the same, brain response differed when the shocks occurred predictably or unpredictably. In particular, the area of the brain that deals with sustained fear responses (the *bed nucleus* of the *stria terminalis*) was *only* activated during unpredictable threats. The researchers concluded that anticipating unpredictable threats—such as fibro flares—often leads to an increase in sustained anxiety and fear because of activation of these specific regions in the brain.

In another experiment, published in the journal *Pain*, perceived pain intensity also increased with unpredictability. Poor predictability of when a shock might be received increased arousal of the nervous system, fear, and perceived pain severity. Receiving shocks in an unpredictable pattern resulted in people rating their pain approximately one point higher on a 1–10 pain scale, where 0 equals no pain and 10 equals severe pain.

The unpredictability of fibromyalgia symptoms can also lead to problems with concentration, memory, and thinking—often called *fibro fog*. Scientists at the University of Texas Health Center studied the effects of chronic unpredictable stress on the intellectual functions of laboratory rats. They found that rats exposed to chronic and unpredictable stress did poorly in experiments that tested their ability to investigate and make decisions, compared to rats that were not exposed to unpredictable stresses.

Chronic, unpredictable stress affects our ability to think, plan, and organize. The unpredictable nature of fibromyalgia may contribute to fibro fog.

SUMMARY

- ▶ Fibromyalgia is a painful condition of the muscles and connective tissue.
- ▶ It affects both men and women, and can occur at any age, although it most often begins in young adulthood or middle age.
- ▶ The most common symptoms are pain, poor sleep, and fatigue, but fibromyalgia can also cause stiff joints, weakness, headaches, bowel

and bladder symptoms, sore eyes, dizziness, depression or anxiety, and difficulty breathing. These symptoms can be unpleasant, disabling, and unpredictable.

▶ Fibromyalgia is sometimes referred to as an "invisible" disability, because a person with this condition can look completely normal.

Who Gets Fibromyalgia and What Should I Expect?

As with many chronic pain syndromes, fibromyalgia is more common in women, although men, children, and adolescents can also develop it. Fibromyalgia affects many aspects of daily life and family relationships, although the primary impact is on the quality of life for the person with the condition. Fibromyalgia also affects a person's ability to participate fully in work and a career but, fortunately, the symptoms of fibromyalgia can be controlled with appropriate treatment.

FIBROMYALGIA IS MORE THAN A YOUNG WOMAN'S DISEASE

Fibromyalgia affects women and men in all age groups. Although fibromyalgia symptoms often start in younger women, they don't go away with age.

ISN'T FIBROMYALGIA AN ADULT'S DISEASE?

Studies fairly consistently show that approximately 1 percent of children and adolescents have fibromyalgia. As in adults, children and ado-

Fibromyalgia affects approximately 1 in 100 children and adolescents, usually beginning around 13–14 years of age. lescents with fibromyalgia also experience problems with fatigue, poor sleep, anxiety, headaches, numbness, and other complaints. The *good* news for children and adolescents with fibromyalgia is that they tend to do better than adults who develop fibromyalgia.

WILL FIBROMYALGIA GO AWAY AFTER MENOPAUSE?

A survey of 100 women with fibromyalgia found that the average woman started experiencing fibromyalgia symptoms at age 46, and menopause had already occurred before fibromyalgia started in two of three women. (In Westernized cultures, menopause is generally expected to occur around age 51.) Although doctors don't know why, studies consistently show that menopause tends to occur earlier in women with fibromyalgia—around age 42.

Women with fibromyalgia start menopause nearly 10 years earlier than average. When fibromyalgia starts before menopause, it generally continues after it. The decade between the ages of 55 and 65 has the highest percentage of affected women. So, unlike other painful conditions (such as migraine) that often lessen with menopause, for many women, fibromyalgia symptoms continue into their senior years.

I THINK MY HUSBAND HAS FIBROMYALGIA

Although fibromyalgia is more common in women, men can also be affected. Because fibromyalgia is generally thought of as a "woman's disease," it's often harder for a man to get diagnosed with fibromyalgia. An interesting study conducted at George Washington University and pub-

GET THE FACTS ON FIBROMYALGIA IN CHILDREN AND ADOLESCENTS

What You Should Know	Here's the Evidence
How many children have fibromyalgia?	Approximately 1 in 100 children and adolescents
When does fibromyalgia usually start?	Most start having symptoms when they're approximately 13–14 years old
What are the most common fibromyalgia symptoms in children and adolescents?	Aching all over, headaches, and problems with sleep occur in most young people with fibromyalgia. Approximately one in four have stiffness or swelling, and one in five complain of fatigue.
What happens with fibromyalgia in youths?	During an average follow-up time of over 18 months, symptoms improved for two of every three children with fibromyalgia. In most cases, kids whose symptoms were improving had followed an aerobic exercise program.
What treatments are used to treat fibromyalgia in children?	Few studies have tested which treatments work in children with fibromyalgia. Educating children and their parents, getting involved in regular aerobic exercise, and learning cognitive behavioral therapies* are effective for reducing pain, disability, and time lost from school. The number of studies to test the use of medications in young people has been limited because of concerns about side effects. Thus, treatment should focus initially on effective non-drug therapies.

*Cognitive behavioral therapies include changing attitudes about the symptoms of fibromyalgia and behaviors caused by the symptoms, learning relaxation techniques, and using techniques to distract oneself from pain, such as walking or exercising. These techniques are discussed in detail in Chapter 7.

lished in the journal *Gender Medicine* found that doctors who specialize in treating conditions such as fibromyalgia are less likely to diagnose it in men, often requiring more physical findings before they make the

Fibromyalgia is less common in men, and it's harder for men to get a fibromyalgia diagnosis from their doctors.

diagnosis than are required for women with the same symptoms. Among fibromyalgia symptoms, men tend to have fewer tender points and less fatigue than women.

As with most medical conditions, men with fibromyalgia typically delay seeing a physician until their symptoms are serious and disability has developed. The good news for men with fibromyalgia is that, when they do finally see a doctor, they can expect the same positive results from non-drug treatments as can women. While most medications also are similarly effective for men and women, the antidepressant duloxetine (Cymbalta®) has shown good effectiveness for women but not for men.

FIBROMYALGIA AFFECTS EVERYDAY LIFE AND FAMILY

Fibromyalgia can have a profound impact on everyday life. A national survey of women with fibromyalgia reported in the journal *Women's Health Issues* found that:

- ► Two in five women with fibromyalgia had difficulty doing heavy household chores, such as cleaning floors, vacuuming, or raking leaves.
- ► One in three had difficulty carrying a bag of groceries.
- ► One in four had difficulty shopping.
- ► Climbing stairs was a substantial problem for one in four women.
- ► One in five had a significant problem walking one or two blocks.

Women with fibromyalgia often worry that their symptoms will disrupt family life when they are unable to fulfill the physical, social, and emotional needs of others in the household. Missing important family events, such as a child's soccer game or a school play, can lead to frustration for both the person with fibromyalgia and other family members. However, having a family member with fibromyalgia doesn't result in a significant overall burden on others in the family. A small study published in the journal *Rheumatology International* in 2011 compared people with fibromyalgia to healthy adults and found that problems with pain, fatigue, poor sleep, and loss of libido were *not* increased in relatives living with a family member who had fibromyalgia. The researchers concluded that living with someone with fibromyalgia does not cause significant health complaints, emotional distress, or reduced quality of life.

Living with someone who has fibromyalgia does not result in significant emotional distress or poor quality of life.

One recent study from Indiana and Purdue Universities suggested that women with fibromyalgia do need to be aware that their symptoms may be affecting their marriage. The study compared marital satisfaction in husbands of women with fibromyalgia and a similar group of husbands of healthy women. Both groups had been married an average of 26 years. Although marital satisfaction was within the normal range for both groups, satisfaction was significantly lower among the spouses of women with fibromyalgia. Dissatisfaction was based on lack of social support and strain in domestic roles and sexual relationships, indicating that those with fibro must be sensitive to the burden the disease places on their spouses and make sure their needs are also being met.

FIBROMYALGIA AFFECTS WORK AND CAREERS

Fibromyalgia often affects the ability to work. A survey comparing people with fibromyalgia to individuals being treated for other conditions found that 47 percent of those with fibromyalgia had lost a job because of the disease, compared with only 14 percent of people losing a job for

THE KEY DIFFICULTIES REPORTED BY PEOPLE WITH FIBROMYALGIA

Physical Symptoms	Mental Symptoms	Social Difficulties	Work Difficulties
Pain	Depression	Disrupted family relationships	Reduced daily activities
Fatigue	Anxiety	Social isolation	Reduced leisure time
Poor sleep	Poor concentration	Disrupted relationships with friends	Limiting physical activities
	Disorganized thinking		Loss of career or career advancement
	Memory problems		

Be sure to talk to your doctor about your fibromyalgia symptoms. You might try circling those items that trouble you and then share this list with your doctor. Be sure to write in any additional concerns.

another health problem. In another survey, people with fibromyalgia lost three times as many workdays as compared to healthy workers.

WHY DID I GET FIBROMYALGIA AND HOW CAN I MAKE IT GO AWAY?

In most cases, people don't know why their fibromyalgia started. The symptoms of fibromyalgia begin for approximately two in five people after an injury or trauma. A report published in the journal *Rheumatology* linked trauma from surgery and work injuries with fibromyalgia. Interestingly, fibromyalgia beginning after an injury tends to cause greater pain, disability, and emotional distress than fibromyalgia that begins with no obvious causal link.

Fibromyalgia may have been passed to you through your family. Recent studies suggest a strong family link with fibromyalgia. Studies

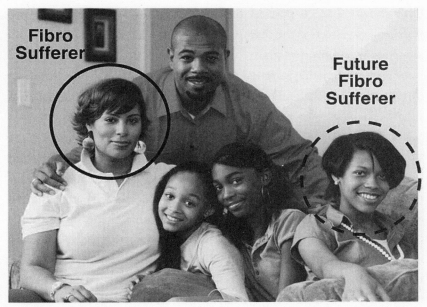

Approximately one in three children of a woman with fibromyalgia will likely develop the condition.

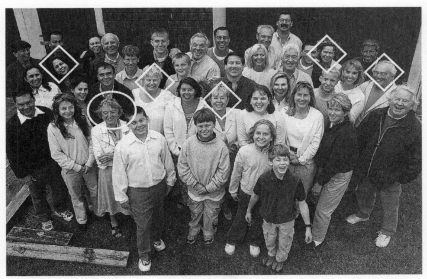

Fibromyalgia runs in families: Aunt Mae has fibromyalgia (circled), and so do approximately one-quarter of her blood relatives (diamonds).

have shown that 28 percent of people born to a mother who had fibromyalgia also had the disease, as did 26 percent of blood relatives of someone with fibromyalgia.

Some people have argued that you don't inherit a susceptibility to fibromyalgia, but rather that you learn to talk about having pain all over your body when you grow up in a family in which other people talk about widespread pain. This argument was debunked by a large study that evaluated fibromyalgia in relatives of people with two different types of chronic widespread pain. They looked at 533 relatives of people with fibromyalgia and 272 relatives of people with rheumatoid arthritis. Among the relatives they were able to interview, fibromyalgia could be diagnosed in 19 percent of those with an affected relative and in only 4 percent of those related to someone with rheumatoid arthritis. So, if you have a relative with fibromyalgia, you're over eight times more likely to also have fibromyalgia yourself than if your relative had rheumatoid arthritis.

WHAT HAPPENS NEXT?

Unlike people with many other medical conditions, people with fibromyalgia have a good understanding about what to expect. A survey of almost 200 people with fibromyalgia found that they correctly understood the following:

- ▶ Fibromyalgia symptoms will likely be chronic.
- ▶ The symptoms are expected to fluctuate over time.
- ▶ Fibromyalgia has a severe impact on physical, social, and psychological functioning.
- ▶ People with fibromyalgia can do a lot to help control their symptoms.
- ▶ Medical treatments are likely to be effective in decreasing symptoms.

This understanding makes people with fibromyalgia open to treatment and appropriately hopeful that they can expect improvement. Unlike some other groups of people with chronic pain, those with fibromyalgia generally don't let negative emotions such as anger affect them.

Are people with fibromyalgia justified in being hopeful about their symptoms? Absolutely! A 5-year study following symptoms in almost 300 women found significant improvement over time in fatigue, function, and depression. Improvement occurred after 1 year, with greater improvement over the following 4 years. So, the good news is that there's light at the end of the tunnel. The bad news is that the tunnel is long—improvement will occur, but it's probably not going to happen overnight, after a few weeks, or even after a few months.

THE GOOD NEWS ABOUT FIBROMYALGIA

Although no one wants to have fibromyalgia, it's important to remember that getting the correct diagnosis does have some positive aspects.

Fibromyalgia Is a Real, Biological Condition

You're not the only one who has these unpleasant, sometimes strange, and often changing symptoms. As you'll read in Chapter 5, an explosion of research has been looking into the causes of fibromyalgia. Although scientists still do not know exactly why fibromyalgia occurs, their research clearly shows that fibromyalgia is real and that it's linked to abnormalities in pain processing in the nerves and other tissues.

Fibromyalgia Is Not a Degenerative Disease

Fibromyalgia does *not* destroy joints, muscles, or nerves. Although people with fibromyalgia will likely continue to have symptoms for a while after their diagnosis, they will not lose the ability to walk or need to use a walker or wheelchair. Symptoms may be better or worse on different days, but you should not expect to develop other serious problems.

Fibromyalgia Is Treatable

Most people with fibromyalgia *do* get better over time. There's no cure or quick fix, and improvement can take weeks to months—but you can expect improvement. Fortunately, a wide assortment of effective non-drug therapies, prescription medications, and nutritional supplements are available for the management of fibromyalgia. You will need to experiment a bit to find out which treatment or combination of treatments works best for you. Most people use non-drug therapies, such as aerobic exercise and pain management techniques, but medications often are temporarily necessary and helpful in conjunction with non-drug treatments.

WHAT KIND OF DOCTOR SHOULD I SEE FOR FIBROMYALGIA?

Many different types of physicians treat patients with fibromyalgia, including:

▶ Primary care doctors (family physicians or internists)
▶ Rheumatologists
▶ Physiatrists (rehabilitation specialists)
▶ Neurologists
▶ Pain management specialists

Rheumatologists are sometimes considered arthritis specialists. Although fibromyalgia is not a disease of the joints or a type of arthritis, rheumatologists often also specialize in treating it.

In many cases, primary care physicians, including family doctors or internists, can effectively manage the symptoms of fibromyalgia. If your primary care doctor has failed to achieve good results, you may wish to see a rheumatologist or other fibromyalgia or pain specialist. You can find a fibromyalgia specialist in your area by clicking on the "find a specialist" button at the Fibromyalgia Information Foundation website (myalgia.com) and through the "resources" link and "healthcare provider directory" button at the National Fibromyalgia Association webpage (www.fmaware.org).

You can also click on the "providers" button of the National Pain Foundation website (www.nationalpainfoundation.org); type in your location and search "by pain condition," selecting fibromyalgia. If you live near a medical school or university, try contacting their rheumatology or pain management departments and asking for a referral to their fibromyalgia expert.

In many cases, you might also work with other health care professionals who offer effective fibromyalgia treatments. These might include:

▶ Behavioral psychologists—to teach you specific pain management skills
▶ Physical therapists or exercise trainers—to develop and monitor exercise programs and address additional muscle or joint problems
▶ Occupational therapists—to address scheduling, problems with getting tasks done, or issues at work
▶ Nutritionists—to address diet, weight management, and the use of herbs and supplements

Don' forget that *you* are the most important member of your health care treatment team. Your health care providers can give you the tools you need to help reduce your fibromyalgia symptoms and the impact these symptoms have on your life, but the success of your treatment depends on your commitment and motivation to incorporate the treatments into your daily life.

WHAT SHOULD I DO BEFORE I SEE MY DOCTOR?

Spend some time thinking about your symptoms, so that you are prepared to answer these questions:

- ► What are two to four of your most troublesome symptoms, and how do they affect you and your daily routine?
- ► What other symptoms do you experience often?
- ► Where do you expect to have pain on different days—which areas of your body?
- ► When did your symptoms first start? Did they start within a short time of having a traumatic injury?
- ► Does anyone else in your family have fibromyalgia or symptoms similar to yours—mom, dad, sisters/brothers, or children?
- ► How many hours do you typically sleep at night? Do you feel rested after sleeping?
- ► Has another doctor diagnosed you with fibromyalgia? Do you know what tests were ordered?
- ► What has been done in the past to treat your fibromyalgia?
- ► Do your symptoms interfere with work or school, or cause you to miss out on family activities?
- ► Do you have other medical conditions or health symptoms?
- ► What medications (over-the-counter, prescription, and natural remedies/supplements/vitamins) do you use? What do you take when you have a fibro flare?

Answers to these questions will help your doctor make the proper diagnosis and start designing your individualized treatment program.

WHAT TO EXPECT FROM YOUR
VISIT TO THE DOCTOR

Don't expect to get all of your questions answered in one visit. You will probably need to work with your health care provider over several visits to refine your particular fibromyalgia treatment strategy. You should expect to learn the answers to these questions:

▶ Do I have fibromyalgia? Has my doctor made sure another problem is not causing my symptoms?
▶ Do I need further testing?
▶ Is my health care provider comfortable treating fibromyalgia?
▶ What can I start doing to reduce my symptoms? Where should I start making changes in my life?
▶ Will I need to take medication?
▶ Are there treatments that can relieve my symptoms without medication?
▶ What if I become pregnant?
▶ Where can I learn more about fibromyalgia?
▶ When should I see the doctor again?

You will find general answers to many of these questions throughout this book, and your health care provider can help clarify what you might expect in your individual situation.

SUMMARY

Fibromyalgia is a real, biological condition with complex and variable symptoms and abnormalities throughout the body. Fibromyalgia also:

▶ Tends to run in families
▶ Is not a degenerative condition

▶ Affects 2–3 percent of adults and 1 percent of children
▶ Has no cure, although effective treatments are available to help make symptoms less severe and to reduce their interference in daily life
▶ Affects three times as many women than men

Part II

Fibromyalgia Symptoms and The Science Behind the Disease

Fibromyalgia is a complex disorder with a wide variety of disabling symptoms. How can one disorder cause problems with pain, sleep, the digestive system, the bladder, and more? This assorted collection of symptoms is probably part of the reason why it took doctors so long to recognize that fibromyalgia was, in fact, a single disorder.

The symptoms characteristic of fibromyalgia could be the result of the abnormalities in physiology that scientists have uncovered in people with this condition. Doctors have not yet discovered what specifically causes fibromyalgia, but they have identified a number of important changes in the body that can explain at least some of the symptoms. Changes in nerves and muscles probably influence pain levels and weakness. Hormonal changes may result in other common symptoms; for example, abnormal melatonin levels may cause sleep problems, and thyroid deficiencies may affect mood and fatigue.

As scientists learn more about fibromyalgia, research is helping convince people with fibromyalgia and their doctors that fibromyalgia is a real, biological condition. This increased understanding has also helped experts develop new systems for identifying and diagnosing fibromyalgia. Increasing knowledge about the genetics and underlying physiology of fibromyalgia will help improve the ability to diagnose and treat this complex condition.

Fibromyalgia Is More
Than Just Pain

Fibromyalgia is considered to be a *chronic pain condition*, but pain is only one of the many troublesome symptoms women with fibromyalgia are likely to experience. In many cases, pain is not their worst difficulty.

In a survey of almost 2,600 people with fibromyalgia—97 percent of whom were women—approximately two in five identified the following problems:

- ► Pain:
  - Low back pain
  - Headaches
  - Arthritis
  - Muscle spasm
- ► Sleep and tiredness:
  - Chronic fatigue
- ► Digestive issues:
  - Irritable bowel syndrome
  - Bloating
- ► Emotional distress:
  - Depression
  - Anxiety

► Nervous system problems:
- Balance difficulties
- Numbness
- Tingling

Some people may find that one or two symptoms really bother and limit them. Others are affected by pain in many parts of their bodies. Sometimes, fibromyalgia involves having pain, feeling exhausted, and being afraid that your next meal will set off a bout of diarrhea. Others may be worn out by a combination of pain, not being able to get a good night's sleep, and constant anxiety.

It's important to discuss each of the symptoms you experience with your doctor, for two reasons. First, although each of these symptoms is common in fibromyalgia, each can also occur as the result of other medical conditions. Your doctor may refer to these symptoms as *non-specific*, meaning that you can experience them with fibromyalgia, as well as with a wide variety of other health conditions. Therefore, it's important to make sure you don't have another illness before treating your symptoms as part of fibromyalgia. Second, your doctor will want to tailor your individual fibromyalgia treatment to target your most severe symptoms. Some treatments help a broad range of fibromyalgia symptoms; others are more effective for individual symptoms.

Be sure your doctor understands your full range of symptoms. Although many, most, or all of them may be part of your fibromyalgia, many of the same difficulties can occur with other health conditions.

"I CAN'T REMEMBER THE LAST TIME I GOT A GOOD NIGHT'S SLEEP."

Poor sleep is a common complaint for women with fibromyalgia. Before we can really understand poor sleep, we have to first understand

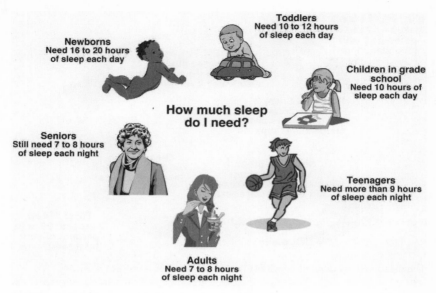

Healthy sleep requirements change over your lifetime.

normal, healthy sleep. Sleep needs change over a lifetime. You often hear people say that the older you get, the less sleep you need. That's only true when you're a child. Once you become an adult, you continue to need 7–8 hours of sleep each night—even as you grow older.

What Is Normal Sleep?

Sleep can be divided into rapid eye movement (REM) sleep when you have dreams, and sleep during which your eyes don't move, called non-REM sleep. The deeper stages of non-REM sleep are also referred to as *restorative sleep*. Healthy adults who sleep 8 hours a night will spend approximately 6 hours in non-REM sleep and 2 hours in REM sleep.

Sleep generally occurs by moving through a series of stages, starting with the lightest: Stage 1 of non-REM sleep; moving to deeper stages of non-REM sleep; and, finally, to REM, or dream, sleep. It's easy to be roused during the lighter stages of sleep. If you wake up during Stage 1, you'll probably feel as if you haven't slept at all. This is often the stage

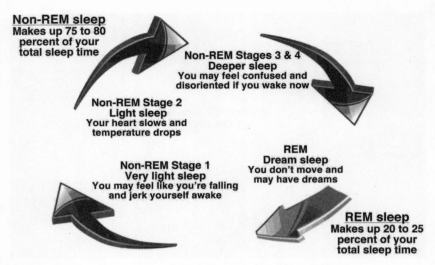

The sleep cycle is divided into REM and four stages of non-REM sleep.

people experience when they fall asleep in front of the television. When you wake them up, they might say, "I wasn't sleeping. I was just resting my eyes."

Sleepwalking can occur during the deep sleep you experience before REM sleep. Once you're in dream sleep, you can no longer move. Some experts believe this temporary paralysis during dream sleep is the body's natural defense to keep people from acting out their dreams while they are asleep.

In general, people spend approximately 90 minutes in non-REM sleep before REM sleep begins. They continue to move through this cycle of light, to deep, to REM sleep, and back to light sleep again throughout the night. You may hear people say, "I was in a deep sleep all night," but everybody actually shifts between light and deep sleep several times each night.

As we get older, our sleep patterns change because of changes in brain chemicals, such as cortisol, growth hormone, and melatonin. These chemical changes cause us to spend more time in the less restful, lighter stages of sleep, and less time in the deeper stages 3 and 4 of non-REM sleep. That's why, as you get older, you may notice you wake up more easily and more frequently at night, and have a harder time falling back to sleep. Because your sleep is less restful, it's especially important that you don't shortchange yourself on total sleep hours.

Do I Really Need to Sleep?

Why do we need to sleep? No one really knows the full answer to this age-old question. What we *do* know is that sleep is essential to good health. During sleep, there are important shifts in a wide range of chemicals in the body, including those that regulate blood sugar and metabolism, hormones important for immune system function, and brain chemicals such as catecholamines. The catecholamines are "fight-or-flight" substances that include epinephrine, norepinephrine, and dopamine, which are also important pain messengers. Poor sleep has been linked to an increased risk for several serious health problems:

▶ Poor sleep increases the inflammatory chemicals that, in turn, increase the risk of arthritis, diabetes, high blood pressure, and heart disease.

▶ Sleep is nature's appetite suppressant, and people who don't sleep enough are more likely to become overweight and obese.

Poor Sleep Lowers Your Pain Threshold

Poor sleep also lowers your pain threshold, both making you more sensitive to pain and making your pain more intense. It's easy to see how not sleeping and feeling a bit crabby can make you tolerate your pain less well. But there's more to it than that. Sleep seems to directly affect how the brain experiences sensations as painful or not.

In an interesting experiment with healthy adults who didn't have pain problems, researchers from the Henry Ford Health System measured how hot something had to be before heat was felt as pain. During the experiment, some people were allowed to spend a full 8 hours in bed

Insufficient or poor quality sleep makes you more sensitive to pain. at night—others were only allowed 4 hours. Their sleep stages were carefully monitored to see who might be experiencing disrupted sleep because of abnormal sleep cycles. The pain threshold measured the next day dropped by one-fourth when people had only been allowed to sleep 4 hours the night before. In addition, the pain threshold dropped by one-third when people had disrupted sleep, with an abnormal cycling of non-REM and REM sleep. These experiments clearly show that not sleeping enough or having poor quality sleep makes you more sensitive to pain.

Do Other People with Fibromyalgia Also Complain About Poor Sleep?

Poor sleep is common in people with fibromyalgia. In one survey, sleep problems were experienced by 81 percent of people with fibromyalgia, compared with only 32 percent of adults without fibromyalgia. Another study comparing sleep problems in over 2,100 people with fibromyalgia, compared to adults in the general population, found that:

▶ Sleep problems and sleepiness scores were over twice as high in people with fibromyalgia.
▶ Scores for achieving adequate sleep were three times higher in the general population than in those with fibromyalgia.
▶ Fewer than one in five people with fibromyalgia slept at least 7 hours at night.

It's not just the number of hours spent sleeping that's the problem in fibromyalgia—quality of sleep is the real issue. Fibromyalgia has been linked to a loss of restorative, deep sleep, with less time spent in the deeper stages 3 and 4 of non-REM sleep. The average adult spends 1–2 hours a night in restorative non-REM sleep, but the average person with fibromyalgia spends only 45 minutes in this stage. In addition,

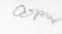

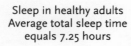

Sleep in healthy adults
Average total sleep time
equals 7.25 hours

Sleep in fibromyalgia
Average total sleep time
equals 6 hours

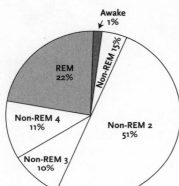

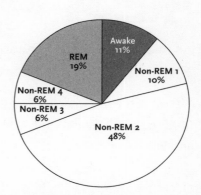

These charts show the percentage of time the average adult spends in the different stages of sleep. Healthy adults sleep longer and almost twice as long in restorative sleep—the deep sleep in non-REM stages 3 and 4—than do those with fibromyalgia.

when healthy people are deprived of restorative sleep, they develop widespread aches and pain, similar to the pain seen in people with fibromyalgia.

"I'M TIRED OF BEING TIRED."

Having poor sleep usually makes people feel tired during the day. Researchers interviewed people with fibromyalgia in the United States and Europe and discovered that:

- ▶ Four in five fibromyalgia patients talked about pain.
- ▶ Two in five talked about fatigue.
- ▶ One in five talked about sleep problems.

When this same group was asked to list their three most troublesome fibromyalgia symptoms, fatigue, tiredness, and lack of energy came in second, after pain, but ahead of disability in daily activities.

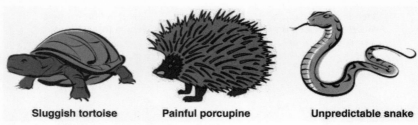

Sluggish tortoise   **Painful porcupine**   **Unpredictable snake**

What animal best represents fibromyalgia?

When this same group was asked, "What animal best represents fibromyalgia?," the top choices highlighted the important role of fatigue and low energy:

- ► Half picked a tortoise or sloth because of low energy.
- ► One in three picked an animal that symbolizes pain, such as a porcupine with spines or a lion with a fierce roar.
- ► One in five picked an animal they considered to be unpleasant *and* unpredictable, such a snake, "because you never know where and when it's going to strike."

Feeling fatigued can also be a problem, even when you sleep well. A study published in the *Journal of the American Academy of Nurse Practitioners* found that over half of women with fibromyalgia whose sleep was disrupted reported moderate or severe fatigue. Nearly one in five of the women with fibromyalgia whose sleep recording monitors showed that they had normal sleep also had moderate or severe fatigue. One in four women who slept well reported moderate to severe problems with energy, and one in 16 women had moderate to severe sleepiness. Another study published in *BMC Musculoskeletal Disorders* found that 40 percent of fibromyalgia patients reported the following:

- ► Feeling fatigued even after a good night's sleep
- ► Having difficulty "getting going" in the morning
- ► Being overwhelmed by their fatigue
- ► Needing to take longer to accomplish tasks because of fatigue

So, when you tell the doctor you're sleeping well but you still feel sleepy and tired, and you have no energy—you're not alone.

What Is Chronic Fatigue Syndrome?

Chronic fatigue syndrome (CFS) describes a medical condition that involves severe fatigue lasting at least 6 months that can't be explained by other health problems or depression. People with CFS also complain of typical fibromyalgia symp-

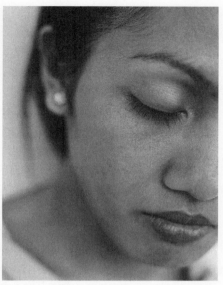

People with fibromyalgia often report having low energy and feeling tired—even when they are getting enough sleep.

toms, including pain, sleep problems, and poor concentration or a clouded memory. Chronic fatigue syndrome affects approximately 2 percent of adults in the United States, Europe, and South America.

Many experts consider feeling sick or exhausted after exercise—called *post-exertional malaise* or *fatigue*—to be a key feature of CFS. Often these symptoms last for 24 hours or longer after completing exercise. In some cases, post-exercise fatigue may not begin until a day or more after exercise. Criteria adopted in Canada consider fatigue, post-exertional malaise or fatigue, sleep disturbance, and pain to be the key features of CFS. Furthermore, a study published in 2011 in *Rehabilitation Psychology* found post-exertional malaise to be the most important factor for identifying people with CFS.

Researchers at the Faculty of Physical Education and Physiotherapy in Belgium reported increases in both fatigue and pain after a walking exercise in people with CFS. Furthermore, pain increase was also still noted 24 hours after exercise. Although exercise is typically

SYMPTOMS OF CHRONIC FATIGUE SYNDROME

ALL of the Following	AT LEAST FOUR of These	NONE of the Following
Fatigue that is severe and disabling	Problems with short-term memory or concentration	Another medical problem that causes your fatigue
You have had fatigue for at least 6 months, but not your whole life	Recurring sore throat	Major depression
Fatigue is not caused by exertion and does not get better by simply resting	Tender lymph nodes in your neck or arm pits	Drug or alcohol abuse
	Muscle aches and pains	Severe obesity
	Joint aches without swollen joints	
	A new or different headache	
	Non-refreshing sleep	
	Feeling sick or exhausted after exercise	

expected to increase the levels of pain-relieving chemicals, such as endorphins, in healthy individuals, research by Whiteside and colleagues showed that pain thresholds actually decreased with exercise in people with chronic fatigue. This study suggests that these people have an abnormal biological response to exercise, resulting in increased perceptions of and sensitivity to pain and fatigue and, consequently, symptoms such as post-exertional malaise or fatigue.

Chronic fatigue syndrome may occur in people with fibromyalgia. A survey published in the *Archives of Internal Medicine* found that four in five people seeing a doctor for a diagnosis of CFS could additionally be diagnosed with fibromyalgia. One in five also had CFS. So, even if your main difficulty is fatigue, you might also have fibromyalgia.

Research from the University of Tokyo found that people with fibromyalgia who also had CFS were more likely to have problems shifting between the different stages of sleep, further adding to sleep disruption and a feeling of having unrefreshing sleep. It's important to address all of the symptoms occurring with fatigue, including those associated with pain and sleep issues.

"I Feel As If I'm in a Fog."

Problems with concentration, attention, memory, and being able to plan and complete tasks are commonly seen in people with fibromyalgia. These symptoms are also referred to as *fibro fog*, a term that describes a feeling of being stuck in a cloud that limits a person's ability to perform mental tasks. People often find they have difficulty with multitasking, they feel mentally overloaded, or they are unable to complete mental tasks as quickly as they used to or think they should.

Doctors have started taking these complaints seriously and are investigating what's really happening when people say they have fibro fog. Physicians at Rush Medical College who catalogued cognitive difficulty in people with fibromyalgia found that:

▶ 70 percent reported a drop in memory.
▶ 56 percent reported feeling mental confusion.
▶ 40 percent noticed problems with speech.
▶ 50 percent experienced *both* a drop in memory and confusion.
▶ One in three had problems with memory, confusion, and speech.

They defined fibro fog as a problem with memory combined with confusion. People experiencing fibro fog had 65 percent higher scores for pain, fatigue, and stiffness, compared to people with fibromyalgia who were not experiencing fibro fog.

Objective tests support what people with fibromyalgia report with regard to fibro fog. The

Difficulties with short-term memory and confusion, also called fibro fog, *affects approximately half of all people with fibromyalgia.*

EVALUATING MEMORY IN FIBROMYALGIA		
Mental Task Often Impaired in People with Fibromyalgia	**Description**	**Examples**
Working short-term memory	Memory over approximately 30 seconds combined with another mental task	Doing mental arithmetic
Episodic long-term memory	Remembering specific events	Remembering items on a grocery list
Semantic memory	Recalling facts	Playing word or trivia games
Attention	Focusing on one thing when there are other distractions	Being able to multitask

simple memory tests that doctors perform in their offices won't identify these problems, but they can be documented by neuropsychological testing, which involves an in-depth battery of psychological tests.

Researchers from the University of Michigan compared what people with fibromyalgia said about their memory and how well they performed on detailed memory testing. This important study showed that people with fibromyalgia are good judges of their memory function, and that they don't need sophisticated neuropsychological tests to know they have fibro fog.

"I'M SO IRRITATED AND IRRITABLE."

Any chronic health problem can make you feel frustrated, irritable, and moody. If you're sleeping poorly and feeling exhausted, your mood will likely be worse. Some people are reluctant to mention mood problems to their doctor, perhaps because they think it's normal or because they expect to feel anxious and depressed if they have pain and sleep problems. Maybe you're embarrassed that you snap at your children and cry easily. Perhaps you're afraid that if you tell your doctor you're in a bad mood, your fibromyalgia symptoms will be blamed on depression.

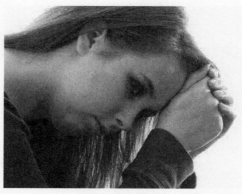

Most people with fibromyalgia feel frustrated, blue, and worried, which can make it more difficult to follow through with fibromyalgia treatments. Be sure to let your doctor know when you are feeling moody.

You are not alone. One in three people with fibromyalgia experiences significant depression or anxiety. It's important for you to know, however, that fibromyalgia is definitely *not* a psychiatric, psychological, or mental health problem. Indeed, research shows that pain and mood problems are not directly related to each other in people with fibromyalgia. They are separate symptoms that do not go hand-in-hand—your pain won't automatically get better just because your mood improves, and vice versa. Mood problems are just one of the many sets of symptoms that often occur in people with fibromyalgia.

Understanding Self-Efficacy and Locus of Control

Self-efficacy is the feeling that you can successfully manage problems and achieve goals. People with fibromyalgia who have a strong sense of self-efficacy have less pain and disability. How well you believe that you can take care of your problems, including fibromyalgia, can also be described by the term *locus of control*. You have a strong *internal* locus of control if you believe that your actions help control how your symptoms will affect you. People with a strong internal locus of control tend to take good care of themselves, stick with healthy lifestyle habits, and

How Do I Know If I Have Depression?

▶ Do you frequently feel sad, irritable, or quick to anger?

▶ Have you stopped enjoying your hobbies and other things you used to enjoy?

▶ Do you feel guilty or hopeless, or worry too much?

▶ Do you feel out of energy or just prefer to sit alone more than usual?

▶ Have you stopped participating in social events with your family or friends?

▶ Are you sleeping too long or having trouble getting to sleep?

▶ Have you experienced an unintentional 10-pound change in your weight?

▶ Do you have thoughts of suicide or death?

Talk to your doctor if you answered "yes" to the last question, or "yes" to at least two of the others. These feelings can be symptoms of depression. They can also be caused by other health problems, such as anemia, thyroid disease, medication side effects, or other medical conditions.

How Do I Know If I Have Anxiety?

▶ Do you frequently worry?

▶ Do you have trouble feeling relaxed? When you try to relax, does your mind start racing about small problems?

▶ Do you have difficulty sitting still or concentrating?

▶ Are you afraid to make a decision and tend to second-guess your choices?

▶ Do groups of people make you nervous or cause you to avoid social situations?

▶ Do you have problems with your stomach or bowel habits?

If you answered "yes" to at least two of these questions, talk to your doctor. These feelings can be symptoms of an anxiety disorder. They can also be caused by other health problems, including low blood sugar, thyroid disease, medication side effects, or other medical conditions.

cope

follow their treatment prescriptions. They see health care providers as resources to help guide them in controlling symptoms.

In contrast, people with an *external* locus of control believe their symptoms are controlled by other people or fate, and tend to become hopeless and helpless. They feel as if there is nothing productive they can do to improve their situation. Because you're reading a book about fibromyalgia, you probably have a healthy internal locus of control—wisely understanding that your actions and thoughts can make a significant impact on how fibromyalgia affects you.

Women with fibromyalgia are more likely to attribute their locus of control to powerful others or fate. This tends to result in increased despair, depression, and anxiety. People who assign their locus of control to fate are also less likely to respond to fibromyalgia treatments. Empowering yourself to understand that there *are* things you

THE ROLE OF LOCUS OF CONTROL IN MANAGING FIBROMYALGIA	
Locus of Control	**Belief**
Internal	This is a healthy perspective in which you understand that *you* can substantially impact your symptoms and disability.
Powerful Others	With this locus of control, you believe that how well you do depends on other people, such as your doctors or therapists. When you have a "powerful others" locus of control, you believe there's nothing you can do except wait for your doctor or therapist to give you something or do a treatment to help you. If they're not available, you're just out of luck and have to suffer.
Fate	People with this locus of control believe there's nothing they or their health care providers can do to make their symptoms better. They believe the outcome is ruled by chance or destiny. When you think fate is in charge, you'll probably find yourself spending lots of time sitting around feeling miserable.

can do to influence your symptoms, as well as how much different symptoms affect you, is an important first step in any successful fibromyalgia treatment.

BOWEL PROBLEMS

Digestive complaints are common in fibromyalgia, including:

- ▶ Irritable bowel syndrome in two of five people with fibromyalgia
- ▶ Bloating in two of five
- ▶ Indigestion or heartburn in one of five

Irritable Bowel Syndrome

Irritable bowel syndrome (IBS) causes chronic stomach pain, bloating, and problems with diarrhea and constipation. Other digestive complaints are also common in people with IBS. An international survey of over 40,000 people with this condition found that they experienced

COMMON SYMPTOMS OF IRRITABLE BOWEL SYNDROME	
Symptom	Percentage of People with Irritable Bowel Syndrome Experiencing Each Symptom
Stomach pain	88 percent
Bloating	80 percent
Trapped wind	66 percent
Tiredness	60 percent
Diarrhea	59 percent
Clothing feels too tight	58 percent
Constipation	53 percent
Heartburn	47 percent

bowel problems on average approximately seven times each month, with about two episodes on each day that they experienced symptoms. Each episode lasted approximately 1 hour.

Episodic abdominal pain, bloating, and changing bowel habits can be symptoms of irritable bowel syndrome.

Most people with symptoms of IBS need an evaluation that includes an analysis of stool and blood samples, and a sigmoidoscopy—which is a test in which your doctor inserts a small flexible tube (about the width of a finger) with a small video camera into your rectum to look into the end of your colon. People 50 years and older will probably need to have

How Do I Know If I Have Irritable Bowel Syndrome?

▶ Have you had stomach pain for at least 6 months?

▶ Over the last 3 months, have you had stomach pain at least 3 days each month?

▶ Over the last 3 months, have you noticed *at least two* of the following:

  • Your pain gets better after you have a bowel movement.

  • Your pain occurs when there's a change in how often you have a bowel movement.

  • When your pain occurs, there's a change in the appearance of your stool.

If your answer is "yes" to all three questions, you may have IBS and should have your complaints evaluated by your doctor.

You are most likely to have another cause for your digestive complaints if:

▶ Your digestive complaints began after age 50.

▶ You have unintentionally lost 10 or more pounds.

▶ You have been experiencing fevers.

▶ You have severe diarrhea, or you get diarrhea during the night.

▶ You have blood in your stool.

▶ Someone in your family has had cancer involving the digestive system.

a more complete examination of the colon, called a colonoscopy. This also uses a narrow, flexible tube with a camera to see the entire length of the colon.

Irritable bowel syndrome is consistently associated with increased pain hypersensitivity and fibromyalgia. Approximately two in five people with fibromyalgia have IBS. In addition, approximately one in three people with IBS will also be diagnosed with fibromyalgia.

BLADDER DIFFICULTIES

Bladder or urinary problems may also occur with fibromyalgia, although these have been studied less extensively than bowel problems. The National Institutes of Health recently formed a Multidisciplinary Approach to the Study of Chronic Pelvic Pain Research Network to help better understand the causes of chronic conditions such as unexplained bladder or pelvic pain.

In general, studies show an increased risk for several pelvic or urinary tract problems with fibromyalgia:

▶ Three in five women with fibromyalgia report pelvic pain, including *vulvodynia*—pain of the external female genital organs that make up the opening to the vagina.
▶ One in five have interstitial cystitis, which is unexplained bladder pain and pressure, with a frequent need to urinate and increased pain during urination.
▶ People with interstitial cystitis or unexplained bladder pain are more likely to have fibromyalgia, IBS, or CFS. Half of the people who have unexplained bladder pain will also have at least one of these other conditions.

If you are experiencing pain or other symptoms involving your bladder or genital area, ask your doctor to do a pelvic examination.

Many easily treatable conditions, such as infections, can also cause similar symptoms.

People with fibromyalgia are approximately twice as likely to report sexual difficulties as healthy adults. Among women with fibromyalgia, the most commonly reported sexual dysfunction complaints are decreased sexual desire, decreased sexual arousal, decreased orgasm, and pain with intercourse.

Although less common than bowel complaints, bladder and other genital complaints can also occur with fibromyalgia.

Sexual dysfunction with fibromyalgia has also been linked to increased depression, so be sure to talk about any sexual and mood issues with your doctor.

What Symptoms Do People with Fibromyalgia Most Want to Improve

Doctors often forget to ask their patients what *they* need to feel better. Fibromyalgia expert and rheumatologist Dr. Robert Bennett and his colleagues at Oregon Health & Science University did just that. They asked almost 800 people with fibromyalgia to rank the symptoms they most wanted to see improved after treatment. Ninety-five percent of the people surveyed were women. Although half chose pain as the symptom they most wanted to improve, half chose common fibromyalgia symptoms related to sleep disturbance, fatigue, and fibro fog.

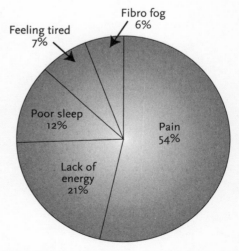

What is the most important symptom people with fibromyalgia want to see improved?

Summary

Fibromyalgia is more than "just pain." For some people with fibromyalgia, other symptoms are just as, or more, disabling. For example:

- ▶ Poor sleep affects four in five people with fibromyalgia, with poor sleep also linked to the increase of pain.
- ▶ Half of those with fibromyalgia experience fibro fog, a term used for memory problems and confusion. These symptoms have been linked to more severe fibromyalgia pain, fatigue, and stiffness.
- ▶ Two in three people with fibromyalgia experience problems with depression or anxiety.
- ▶ Two in five people with fibromyalgia have problems with IBS or bloating.
- ▶ Urinary problems, bladder and genital pain, and sexual dysfunction may also occur in fibromyalgia.
- ▶ Pain, poor sleep, fatigue, and fibro fog are the most important symptoms people with fibromyalgia want to have treated.

4

Fibromyalgia—Is It or Isn't It?
Why Your Doctor Might be
Unsure of Your Diagnosis

As with other chronic pain and medical conditions, many tests are
available to see what you *don't* have when you have fibromyalgia
symptoms. Your doctor can do blood tests, X-rays, and magnetic resonance imaging (MRI scans) to tell you that you *don't* have arthritis,
lupus, infections, or cancer. There's no test, however, that says you *do*
have fibromyalgia.

Years ago, doctors might have told you something like,
"Everything seems normal. All of your tests show that everything's fine.
But if I had to say something, I'd call your condition fibromyalgia."
Luckily, this kind of nonsense is now a thing of the past. Fibromyalgia
specialists have worked hard over the last 20 years—and are continuing
to work hard—to help give doctors specific descriptions and definitions
of fibromyalgia. The diagnosis of fibromyalgia does *not* mean nothing
is wrong. When your doctor tells you that you have fibromyalgia, it
means you have a specific and unique collection of unpleasant symptoms, which you already know all too well.

As you read in Chapter 1, fibromyalgia is a valid medical condition. Even though your bedside tests and basic laboratory studies may
be "normal," detailed testing of your skin, nerves, muscles, and hor-

mones will clearly show that your symptoms have occurred because your body is *not* working normally.

HISTORY OF FIBROMYALGIA

The term *fibromyalgia* is relatively new to medicine. This diagnosis was probably not around when many of your doctors were in medical school. While the term may be new, the cluster of symptoms experienced by people with fibromyalgia has been reported for over 200 years, and several different terms have been used to describe a condition in which

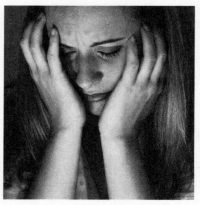

Has your doctor ever told you, "Nothing's really wrong with you; I guess you have fibromyalgia"? Fortunately, the American College of Rheumatology and other organizations are working hard to educate doctors that fibromyalgia is a specific and unique syndrome.

people have had widespread aches and pain, stiffness, sleep disturbance, fatigue, and other symptoms. The medical understanding of fibromyalgia has developed over time:

▶ In the 1800s, physicians called the symptoms of fibromyalgia *muscular rheumatism*. The term *rheumatism* means a problem that affects the joints and surrounding tissues. People with these symptoms didn't develop damaged joints similar to those seen with arthritis, so doctors thought the pain was caused by the way the muscles were affecting the joints.

▶ In 1880, neurologist Dr. George Miller Beard introduced the term *neurasthenia* to describe generalized pain and other symptoms. The term *asthenia* is used to refer to a combination of fatigue, loss of energy, and lack of strength. Dr. Beard thought the nervous system became overwhelmed, with asthenia developing as the result of psychological or emotional distress.

▶ In 1904, English physician Sir William Gowers coined the phrase *fibrositis*. He thought that fibromyalgia symptoms were caused by inflammation. (The medical terms for many inflammatory conditions include the suffix "itis.")

▶ Between 1927 and 1930, three other physicians suggested new terms to highlight what they also believed was a problem associated with inflammation: *myofascitis*, *myofibrositis*, and *neurofibrositis*. *Myo-* means muscles. *Fascia* is the term used for the fibers of connective tissue found throughout the body that help separate the different tissues from each other. Fascia fibers wrap around muscles and form thick bands that connect muscles to bones. *Fibrositis* means an inflammation of fiber tissues.

▶ In 1973, Dr. Essam Awad proposed the term *interstitial myofibrositis* to indicate that a specific disorder of the muscles was not the cause of pain, but rather some kind of inflammation *between* the muscles and connective tissues.

▶ Dr. Philip Hench introduced the term *fibromyalgia* in 1976.

▶ In 1981, Dr. Muhammad Yunus and his colleagues published a controlled study proving that the term *fibromyalgia* described a specific and unique clustering of pain and other symptoms. This landmark study helped doctors begin to understand that fibromyalgia is a specific and unique syndrome.

▶ Fibromyalgia finally gained more widespread credibility in the medical community in 1990, when the American College of Rheumatology established specific classification criteria for the condition. This standard for diagnosing fibromyalgia allowed doctors to better identify patients and helped researchers study this syndrome.

The diagnosis of fibromyalgia has only existed for about 35 years.

▶ In 2010, the American College of Rheumatology proposed a new classification system to diagnose fibromyalgia, one that supports systems used in Europe. This definition may also allow more people to receive an accurate diagnosis of fibromyalgia.

History teaches us two important things about fibromyalgia:

▶ It is a relatively new diagnosis—and your doctor may not be familiar with it.

▶ Doctors are still debating the best way to diagnose fibromyalgia. As a result, one doctor may say you have fibromyalgia, but another may say you don't.

THE FIRST STEP IS FINDING OUT WHAT YOU DON'T HAVE

Fibromyalgia symptoms are *non-specific.* This means that many of the symptoms seen with fibromyalgia are also present in other medical conditions. Your doctor really can't tell you that you have fibromyalgia until he has made certain that you don't have other health issues, some of which are shown in the table.

Before your doctor can diagnose fibromyalgia, you will undergo a thorough evaluation that includes your medical history and current symptoms, and a physical examination. Blood tests are often needed, as well as X-rays and other radiology tests.

MEDICAL CONDITIONS THAT MIMIC FIBROMYALGIA

Bone and Joint Diseases	Autoimmune Disorders	Infections	Hormone Disorders	Cancer
Ankylosing spondylitis	Sjögren's syndrome	Chronic hepatitis C	Diabetes	Multiple myeloma
Osteoarthritis	Systemic lupus erythematosus	Tuberculosis	Thyroid disease	Metastatic cancer
Osteomalacia			Parathyroid disease	
Polymyalgia rheumatica				
Rheumatoid arthritis				

> ## Typical Blood Tests for People with Widespread Pain and Other Symptoms
>
> ▶ Complete blood count
>
> ▶ Tests for inflammation, such as an erythrocyte sedimentation rate or C-reactive protein
>
> ▶ Creatinine kinase
>
> ▶ Blood calcium and vitamin D tests
>
> ▶ Thyroid hormone tests

Changing Criteria for Diagnosing Fibromyalgia

In 1990, the American College of Rheumatology established a widely accepted system for diagnosing fibromyalgia. This system required people to have persistent widespread pain and a number of *tender points*—seemingly unrelated areas on the body that are painful when pressed. Researchers have identified 18 areas that are typically tender when pressed in people who have fibromyalgia.

Don't become frustrated if it takes time to receive a diagnosis. A good doctor will make certain you don't have other health problems that need specific treatment before determining that you have fibromyalgia.

People with fibromyalgia often find the tender point examination a little silly, and may ask their doctors, "But doesn't *everyone* find these spots tender when you press them?" The answer to this is a resounding "no!" At the University of Pittsburgh, we helped develop the tender point examination and studied these areas in people with fibromyalgia and other severe chronic pain conditions. We found that experiencing tenderness when these point areas were pressed was specific for fibromyalgia. Having many sensitive tender points occurs in fibromyalgia, but not in people with pain caused by other conditions—

such as muscle pain, pinched nerves, slipped discs, or arthritis. People with other conditions may have several painful tender points, but they usually don't have as many, and they may also have other issues that help distinguish their symptoms from fibromyalgia. The most important message is that people with fibromyalgia have a different pattern of pain than do people with other chronic pain conditions.

During a tender point examination, the doctor will firmly press each spot in turn with his thumb and ask you if the pressure is painful. Some doctors ask for just a "yes, tender" or "no, just pressure" response. Others may ask you to rate how severe the tenderness is, with zero equaling just pressure and ten excruciating pain.

Your doctor can use the results of the tender point examination to arrive at two numbers:

▶ The *tender point count*—how many tender points are painful; this number will be between zero and 18.
▶ The *tender point score*—if you rated the severity of each point's tenderness, your doctor can add these scores to get a possible total tender point score, ranging from zero to 180.

You and your doctor can follow changes in your tender point count and score as you go through treatment. These numbers usually decrease, indicating successful treatment.

Original 1990 American College of Rheumatology Criteria for the Classification of Fibromyalgia

▶ The pain has been present for at least 3 months.
▶ The pain is widespread, affecting the trunk, both sides of the body, and areas above and below the waist.
▶ When a doctor does a *tender point* examination, at least 11 of the 18 tested spots are tender.
▶ The pain cannot be explained by another medical condition.

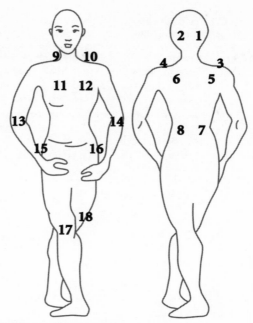

Eighteen Possible Fibromyalgia Tender Points

New Fibromyalgia Diagnostic Criteria Proposed in 2010 and 2011

In 2010 and 2011, the American College of Rheumatology and the Association of the Medical Scientific Societies in Germany each proposed modifying the criteria for diagnosing fibromyalgia. They argued that many physicians don't complete the tender point examination, which means that their patients can't be given a diagnosis of fibromyalgia. In addition, which tender points are positive—and how tender they are—may change on any given day. It is therefore possible that on some days you might have more positive tender points than on others, and on other days you might not have the 11 required tender points. As a result, some people with fibromyalgia may not be diagnosed properly.

Doctors now diagnose fibromyalgia by focusing more on the occurrence of common fibromyalgia symptoms and less on the tender point examination.

THE NEW AMERICAN COLLEGE OF RHEUMATOLOGY PRELIMINARY
FIBROMYALGIA DIAGNOSIS QUESTIONNAIRE

Widespread Pain Index	Symptom Severity Scale	Symptom Severity Scale Supplement
Where do you have pain?	*Rate how severe each of these symptoms has been over the previous week:*	*Have you had these in the last 6 months?*
Shoulder girdle, left	Fatigue	Pain or cramps in the lower abdomen
Shoulder girdle, right	Waking not feeling refreshed	Depression
Upper arm, left	Problems with concentration, memory, or thinking	Headache
Upper arm, right		
Lower arm, left		
Lower arm, right		
Hip or butt, left		
Hip or butt, right		
Upper leg, left		
Upper leg, right		
Lower leg, left		
Lower leg, right		
Jaw, left		
Jaw, right		
Chest		
Abdomen		
Upper back		
Lower back		
Neck		
Scoring: Give yourself 1 point for each region where you feel pain. Possible scores are 0–19.	**Scoring:** Rate each of the following on a scale from 0–3, with zero points for no symptoms: 1 = mild or intermittent symptoms 2 = moderate or often troublesome symptoms 3 = severe, continuous, or disabling symptoms. Add the scores for a possible total score of 0–9.	**Scoring:** Give yourself one point for each symptom you have experienced during the last 6 months for a possible total score of 0–3. Add this number to the Symptom Severity Score for a Total Symptom Severity score.
Score:	Score:	Score:
Pain Score =	Total Symptom Severity Score =	Fibromyalgia-ness score = Pain Score plus Total Symptom Severity Score (possible total score of 0–31)

(This questionnaire can be downloaded from www.diamedicapub.com.)

The two new sets of criteria have added other common symptoms besides pain to help make a diagnosis. Therefore, you might be diagnosed with fibromyalgia even if your doctor doesn't test your tender points, or you don't have the needed 11 tender points on a given day. Regardless of which criteria are used, your doctor needs to complete a thorough examination before the fibromyalgia diagnosis is made to make certain your symptoms are not caused by other health conditions.

You may have fibromyalgia if you have had symptoms of about the same severity for at least 3 months and one of the following based on the new American College of Rheumatology preliminary fibromyalgia diagnosis questionnaire:

▶ A Pain Score of at least 7, and a Total Symptom Severity Score of at least 5
▶ A Pain Score between 3 and 6, and a Total Symptom Severity Score of at least 9
▶ A Fibromyalgia-ness Score of at least 13

ASSOCIATION OF THE MEDICAL SCIENTIFIC SOCIETIES IN GERMANY (AWMF) FIBROMYALGIA DIAGNOSIS QUIZ

If your answer is "yes" to the following questions, you may have fibromyalgia.

Pain

Have you had widespread pain for more than 3 months?

Does the pain affect your trunk, both arms, and both legs?

Complaints Over the Previous 3 Months

Do you have problems with sleep?

Do you have problems with fatigue?

Do you have feelings of swelling or stiffness in at least one of these areas—your hands, feet, or face?

If you answered "yes" to **both of the pain questions** and **all of the complaint questions**, you may have fibromyalgia. You should see your doctor for a complete evaluation and diagnosis.

Take this questionnaire to your doctor for a complete evaluation to see if you have fibromyalgia, or if your symptoms might be caused by another condition.

You might want to complete both of these fibromyalgia questionnaires to see whether your answers suggest that you might have fibromyalgia. However, they can't tell you for certain that you have fibromyalgia—you will need to take the questionnaire(s) to your doctor for a thorough evaluation. The questionnaires can provide a great opening to talk to your doctor about *all* of the symptoms you may be having—both pain and non-pain symptoms.

WHY DID IT TAKE SO LONG TO GET A DIAGNOSIS?

If you feel that it has taken forever to get diagnosed with fibromyalgia, you're not alone. A study published in *BMC Health Services Research* found that it takes over 2 years for most people to get a diagnosis. This study evaluated the diagnosis of 800 people with fibromyalgia worldwide, and the results were fairly consistent—so it's not just you, your doctor, or your health insurance. Getting the diagnosis takes a *long* time.

Why *does* it take so long to get diagnosed? Interestingly, delays occur because most people with symptoms wait before they finally see a doctor. Then it takes quite a while to go through the testing process. In the survey described above, they found that:

▶ People did not see a physician until they had symptoms for an average of over 11 months.
▶ Two in five didn't tell their doctor about their symptoms sooner because they were afraid the doctor wouldn't take their complaints seriously.
▶ Once people told their doctors they were having symptoms that might be fibromyalgia, it took an average of almost 2½ years before a diagnosis was made.

▶ The average person with fibromyalgia saw three or four doctors before finally getting a diagnosis.

If you're new to having symptoms that might be fibromyalgia, and it's taking too long to get a diagnosis, don't worry. The first step is to recognize that your symptoms are serious, treatable, and important to discuss with your doctor. While it may take a long time before your doctor is confident that you definitely have fibromyalgia, you should be able to start treatment to improve your health while the process is under way.

SUMMARY

▶ Fibromyalgia is a specific syndrome with a specific diagnosis that describes a unique set of symptoms, including pain.
▶ People with fibromyalgia have tender points throughout the body that are particularly sensitive to being pressed.
▶ Traditionally, a diagnosis of fibromyalgia has required a person to have at least 11 tender points felt as painful.
▶ Proposed changes to standardized criteria for diagnosing fibromyalgia include a focus on non-pain fibromyalgia symptoms, including poor sleep, fatigue, and "fibro fog."
▶ The 2011 criteria for diagnosing fibromyaliga have made it easier for patients to take a survey questionnaire to see if they may have fibromyalgia.

What Causes Fibromyalgia?

What causes fibromyalgia? The short answer is—we don't know. A more complete answer is that we don't know the specific cause, but—as discussed earlier—we do know that fibromyalgia is a real, biological condition. Medical research has identified a number of abnormalities in the nerves, muscles, hormones, and more of people with fibromyalgia.

However, we *don't* know what individual abnormality or combination of abnormalities causes fibromyalgia. In other words, although changes in nerve endings in the skin and muscles are real, do they *cause* fibromyalgia—or do people experience these changes for some other reason? We know what's wrong, just not which abnormality might have started the fibromyalgia process.

Only partly understanding what causes fibromyalgia offers good news and bad news. Although we know fibromyalgia is real, it is hard to cure a condition when we don't understand the specific causes. Doctors and researchers are continuing to unravel the mysteries of fibromyalgia so that one day we will know what dysfunction actually leads to the disease, which will make it easier to both diagnose and treat.

THE BIOLOGY OF FIBROMYALGIA

A variety of factors have been impli-
cated in the pathophysiology of
fibromyalgia, including changes in
the nerves, muscles, and chemicals
that promote inflammation.

Nerves

Research consistently shows that the
nerves of people with fibromyalgia
look and behave differently than
those of normal people. For example,
nerves in the skin of people with

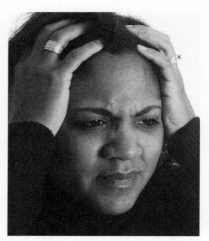

Fibromyalgia is not "all in your head."
Fibromyalgia has been linked to
objective, physiological abnormalities
in nerves, muscles, and some
hormones that may play important
roles in causing fibromyalgia.

fibromyalgia have a different appearance, compared to healthy adults. The
nerve fibers in people with fibromyalgia are smaller in size and lack the
complex folding patterns seen in normal nerves. In addition to looking
different, the nerves of people with fibromyalgia react to pain differently:

▶ People with fibromyalgia have more nerve *receptors*, which are activated by the chemicals that send pain messages to the brain. This
makes it easier for the nerves to identify and send pain signals.

▶ Everyone's skin has many different types of nerve endings. For
example, the nerve endings called *opioid* or *narcotic-type receptors*
react to the body's natural painkillers, called *endorphins*. These opioid receptors function abnormally in people with fibromyalgia.

▶ Specialized magnetic resonance imaging (MRI) scans—used in
research studies to show brain anatomy, function, and metabolism—show subtle but important differences in the areas of the
brain responsible for pain processing in people with fibromyalgia,
compared to healthy adults.

These changes in nerves and in the brain regions related to pain support the increased sensitivity to pain reported by people with fibromyalgia. You may find that you're more sensitive to pain or another symptom that wouldn't bother someone else. This is typical of fibromyalgia, and research evidence proves this sensitivity is not imaginary. It's caused by excitable, overly active nerves that have become more responsive to pain.

Scientists at the Geneva University Hospital in Switzerland tested how well people with fibromyalgia could feel hot and cold, compared to healthy people. There was no difference between the two groups as to when they could first detect that something was hot or cold. This showed that the touch nerves work the same in people with fibromyalgia as in people without the condition. However, as the hot signal got hotter and the cold signal got colder, people with fibromyalgia felt the change in temperature as painful sooner than did those without the disease. This important study further supports the fact that people with fibromyalgia are more sensitive to pain—and that they feel something as painful before others might.

Nerves in the skin and brain are different in people with fibromyalgia, causing them to become more sensitive to pain. This change is called sensitization.

Muscles

There are two types of muscle fibers, type I and type II. You can see the important differences in type I and II fibers in the accompanying table. Type I fibers are used to maintain posture; type II fibers allow us to move around and perform tasks such as lifting heavy objects.

Research studies that tested the muscles of people with fibromyalgia found that type II muscles are smaller than normal in people with fibromyalgia, and they have reduced strength when they contract and less endurance for staying contracted. Scientists speculate that these abnormal type II fibers may cause weakness and fatigue.

Microscopic changes in muscle fibers may explain why fatigue and weakness are common complaints in fibromyalgia.

DIFFERENCES IN TYPE I AND TYPE II MUSCLE FIBERS

Fiber Type	Main Functions	Everyday Example
Type I	Also called *red* fibers or *slow contraction* muscle fibers	Type I fibers make up "dark meat."
	Important for controlling muscle tone and posture	Chicken legs or drumsticks contain more red or type I fibers because the chicken spends most of its time walking slowly.
	Designed to work for long periods of time without tiring	
Type II	Also called *white* fibers or *fast contraction* muscle fibers	Type II fibers make up "white meat."
	Produce strong muscle contractions for short periods of time	Chicken breasts are called "white meat" because they contain mainly white muscle fibers. That's because the chicken only needs to flap its wings for a short period of time to escape from a predator.
	These fibers are more likely to tire with exertion.	If you eat wild birds who spend a lot of time flying and avoiding predators, most of their meat will have mostly red fibers, or be mainly "dark" meat.

IS FIBROMYALGIA INHERITED? WILL MY CHILDREN GET FIBROMYALGIA?

As discussed in Chapter 2, fibromyalgia runs in families. A study published in the journal *Arthritis and Rheumatism* found that you are eight and a half times more likely to have fibromyalgia if you have a relative with fibromyalgia, compared with having a relative with another chronic pain condition such as rheumatoid arthritis.

Scientists are looking for specific genes that might cause fibromyalgia. An article reviewing all of the current gene studies was published in 2011 in the journal *Rheumatology International*. The authors identified three genes that were the most likely to be linked to fibromyalgia.

GENES LINKED TO INCREASED RISK FOR FIBROMYALGIA		
Gene	**Full Name**	**Function**
5-HTTLPR	Serotonin transporter promoter region	Serotonin is a brain chemical that affects pain and mood. Changes in the transporter gene will affect available levels of serotonin.
COMT	Catechol-O-methyl transferase	This is an enzyme that breaks down catecholamines, brain chemicals that are important for pain signaling. Examples of catecholamines include epinephrine, norepinephrine, and dopamine.
5-HT2A	Serotonin 2A receptor	Serotonin is a brain chemical that is important for pain signaling and mood. There are many different areas that respond to serotonin, called receptors. The type 2A receptors are located in the brain and digestive system.

The genes that control the dopamine-D3 receptor have also been linked to fibromyalgia. Researchers from the University of Sherbrooke in Canada evaluated D3 genes and published their findings in the *Journal of Pain*. Although the occurrence of abnormal D3 genes has not been linked to fibromyalgia, individuals with abnormal D3 genes—both people with fibromyalgia and healthy adults—have problems blocking out pain and have a lower heat pain threshold. This indicates that some gene abnormalities—such as those involving dopamine—may be important for pain control for a broader range of problems than just fibromyalgia.

INFLAMMATION AND FIBROMYALGIA

Chemicals in the body called *cytokines* increase inflammation in tissues. They also cause nerves to become more excited and send more pain messages. A group of cytokines called *interleukins*, which play an important role in the body's immune system, have been linked to fibromyalgia. Several research studies have shown abnormally increased levels of several different interleukins in people with fibromyalgia.

A study conducted at Ruprecht-Karls University in Heidelberg, Germany, found that levels of interleukin type 8 were more than twice as high in people with fibromyalgia, compared to the levels expected in healthy adults. After they went through a 3-week, comprehensive treatment program that included education, exercise, and behavioral pain techniques, interleukin-8 levels dropped back to normal levels. This drop in interleukin-8 corresponded to reductions in pain severity.

STRESS AND FIBROMYALGIA

The symptoms of fibromyalgia cannot be entirely explained by stress or a person's reaction to stress. However, stress is an important trigger for aggravating most medical symptoms—including chronic pain. Stress does not *cause* fibromyalgia, but it can certainly make symptoms worse.

Researchers in Tel Aviv investigated the role of stress in chronic widespread pain and other fibromyalgia symptoms by evaluating people living in the Israeli town of Sderot, which experienced repeated missile attacks—and a similar town, Ofakim, which had *not* been attacked. Chronic widespread pain was 45 percent more likely to be experienced by women living in the more stressful Sderot; fatigue and irritable bowel syndrome were also more common. The researchers concluded that the cluster of fibromyalgia-type symptoms were more common in people under chronic stress.

Chronic exposure to stress results in widespread pain, fatigue, and digestive complaints.

We can see and feel our bodies reacting to stress—anger, frustration, worry building, muscles tightening, fists and teeth clenching, and sweating are all common reactions. Stress also causes chemical changes inside us that we may not be aware of, some of which lower our pain threshold and make us more susceptible and sensitive to pain during times of stress. A link between the brain and the adrenal glands, called the *hypothalamic-pituitary-adrenal axis*, is activated when you are under stress. The hypothalamus and the pituitary gland in the brain send messages to the adrenal glands. These messages cause the adrenal glands to release cortisol during times of stress.

Cortisol has been called the "stress hormone." The release of cortisol gives us a quick burst of energy, improved memory, and reduced

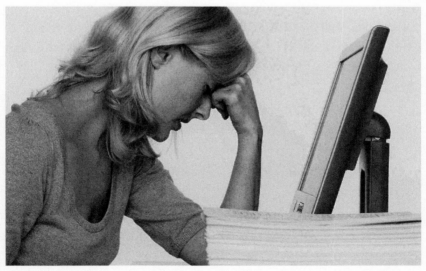

Emotional stress results in a wide range of physical and chemical changes in the body that lower the pain threshold and increase sensitivity to pain.

sensitivity to pain. This important natural survival aid has developed to allow us to more effectively flee from or fight a predator. Cortisol is called the "flight or fight" hormone for this reason. Have you ever had a teacher or boss who made you nervous on purpose and then told you: "People perform better when they are under a bit of stress"? The boost we get from cortisol when stressed is what they are talking about.

Studies on the stress response in people with fibromyalgia were recently reviewed in the journal *Stress*. These studies suggest that the stress response mechanism is less resilient, and the hypothalamus and pituitary gland often don't react as strongly as they should. The cortisol response is also often less than normal. In effect, people with fibromyalgia get all the negatives of stress and none of its temporary benefits. Some experts believe that the body's abnormal biological response to stress is why stress aggravates the symptoms of fibromyalgia.

ABUSE

Abuse comes in many forms—physical violence, emotional abuse, sexual assaults, and neglect. It may be inflicted on children or adults. Unfortunately, abuse is common. The World Health Organization has provided these staggering statistics:

- ▶ A survey of adults in ten countries found that 15–70 percent of women had been physically or sexually abused by a spouse or intimate partner.
- ▶ Twenty-five to 50 percent of people were physically abused as children.
- ▶ Up to 10 percent of men and 20 percent of women were sexually abused as children.

Even if the abuse is no longer occurring, its effects can be long lasting. A survey of nearly 3,400 women in Canada found that victims of physical abuse alone were two and a half times more likely to experience disabling chronic pain. Victims of both physical and sexual abuse were 60 percent more likely to have disabling pain. Studies have also linked both childhood and adult abuse to an increased risk for developing migraines and for more severe migraine patterns. Data from the National Comorbidity Study in the United States also found a 50 percent increased risk for arthritis among victims of childhood abuse.

A study published in *Arthritis Care and Research* found strong links between abuse and fibromyalgia:

▶ You are two and a half times more likely to have fibromyalgia if you were physically abused as a child, and three times more likely if you were physically abused as an adult.

▶ You are twice as likely to have fibromyalgia if you were the victim of sexual abuse as either a child or adult.

Victims of abuse are also at risk for a wide range of other health problems. A study from Columbia University showed increased risks for developing heart disease, lung disease, peptic ulcer disease, diabetes, and autoimmune disorders in victims of childhood abuse. Abuse victims are also at higher risk for developing self-destructive behaviors and post-traumatic stress disorder (PTSD), with flashbacks or nightmares, anxiety, avoidance of reminders of the abuse, and having difficultly connecting closely with others.

One of the best treatments for the effects of abuse, neglect, and PTSD is cognitive-behavioral therapy, in which you work on identifying distressing and dysfunctional patterns of thinking and change them to less destructive ones. Changing your thoughts is often an important first step toward improving behaviors and symptoms. Relaxation techniques and mindfulness meditation can also be helpful. These skills are generally taught by working with a trained psychologist.

The "bottom line" is that abuse you experienced either long ago or recently may be negatively affecting you and those around you. Hiding

THE PRIMARY CARE POST-TRAUMATIC STRESS DISORDER (PTSD) SCREEN*

Has something so frightening, horrible, or upsetting happened to you (recently or some time ago) that you experienced any of the following in the past month?

	YES	NO
Had nightmares about the experience or thought about it when you didn't want to	❏	❏
Tried hard not to think about it or went out of your way to avoid situations that reminded you of it	❏	❏
Felt as if you were constantly on guard, watchful, or easily startled	❏	❏
Felt numb or detached from others, activities, or your surroundings	❏	❏

If you answered "yes" to at least three of these questions, you may have PTSD and you should talk to your doctor.

*Adapted from Prins et al. The primary care PTSD screen (PC–PTSD): Development and Operating Characteristics. *Primary Care Psychiatry* 2003; 9:9–14. Also available online at http://www.ptsd.va.gov/professional/pages/assessments/pc-ptsd.asp

signs of abuse doesn't make its consequences go away. These effects of abuse need to be treated seriously, as with all health problems. It's important to work with a professional who can help you identify how the abuse may still be affecting you and teach you ways take back control of your life. This can be done as you're simultaneously working on other fibromyalgia treatments with your doctor.

To get more information and find a licensed psychologist near you, visit these websites:

▶ American Psychological Association at http://www.apa.org/
▶ Association for Behavioral and Cognitive Therapies at http://www.abct.org/Home/
▶ American Headache Society resources section at http://www.achenet.org/

HORMONES AND FIBROMYALGIA

Hormones are chemical substances that are made by cells in one part of the body and released to affect different cells, often in other parts of the body. Hormones can be stored in organs called *glands* and released later when needed. Your body produces many hormones besides the stress hormone cortisol. These hormones affect growth, development, and reproduction, as well as regulate metabolism, the immune system, and mood.

IMPORTANT HORMONES PRODUCED BY THE BODY

Hormone's Name	Where the Hormone Is Produced	What the Hormone Does
Cholecystokinin	Small intestine	Releases digestive enzymes
Cortisol	Adrenal glands	Regulates blood sugar levels and metabolism of food, blood pressure, inflammation, and the immune system
Erythropoietin	Kidneys	Makes red blood cells
Growth hormone	Pituitary gland	Controls growth
Insulin	Pancreas	Directs metabolism of carbohydrates and fats
Leptin	Fat cells	Manages appetite and fat metabolism
Melatonin	Pineal gland	Controls sleep
Renin	Kidneys	Regulates blood pressure
Sex hormones, such as estrogen, progesterone, and testosterone	Mainly ovaries, testes, and adrenal glands	Regulates reproductive development
Thyroid hormone	Thyroid gland	Adjusts body temperature, heart rate and blood pressure, metabolism, and weight

Hormonal imbalances in people with fibromyalgia help explain possible causes and suggest potential treatments.

Growth and thyroid hormones seem to have the strongest influence on fibromyalgia. Sex hormones, such as estrogen, may also influence the severity of fibromyalgia symptoms.

Melatonin

Melatonin is a hormone produced by the pineal gland in the brain. It plays an important role in controlling sleep cycles, and it has also been linked to blood pressure, mood, the growth of cancer cells, and even the development of Alzheimer's disease. Several studies have examined melatonin levels in women with fibromyalgia. Two studies found that melatonin levels were abnormal in people with fibromyalgia, but two others—including the most recent studies from Harvard Medical School and Brigham and Women's Hospital—failed to find differences in melatonin levels between women with fibromyalgia and healthy, pain-free women. Even though a lack of melatonin has not been consistently reported with fibromyalgia, melatonin supplementation does reduce symptoms, as we will discuss in Chapter 9.

Growth Hormone

The body produces growth hormone during deep sleep stages 3 and 4, the restorative sleep discussed in Chapter 3. When parents tell their children they need to get a good night's sleep to grow, they are absolutely right.

You might think that growth hormone is only important for children. As the name suggests, growth hormone *is* important for controlling a child's growth, but it also plays an important role in adults. Low growth hormone levels in adults result in low energy, difficulties with memory and concentration, and a "blue" mood—many of the same symptoms seen with fibromyalgia.

Growth hormone also causes the release of another hormone, *insulin-like growth factor*, or IGF-1. A low IGF-1 level has been found in approximately one in three people with fibromyalgia. This suggests that an imbalance in growth hormone might be an important factor in the development of fibromyalgia.

Thyroid Hormone

Fibromyalgia and thyroid disease seem to be linked. When our defense mechanisms become misdirected against our own bodies—a process called *autoimmunity*—it can prevent the body from functioning normally. One example is rheumatoid arthritis, in which antibodies attack the tissues of the joints.

Doctors at the University of Pisa found that antibodies against the thyroid gland cause thyroid autoimmunity in approximately two in five people with fibromyalgia. The individuals with thyroid antibodies had more symptoms, including increased pain sensitivity. They also reported in a link between Hashimoto's thyroiditis and fibromyalgia. Hashimoto's thyroiditis is an autoimmune disease in which a person makes antibodies against her own thyroid gland. As a result, the gland makes less and less hormone, causing hypothyroidism. This results in fatigue, depression, weight gain, constipation, vague aches and pains, and other unpleasant symptoms. These researchers believe that autoimmune factors affecting the thyroid may lead to fibromyalgia. Similar to fibromyalgia, Hashimoto's thyroiditis and many other autoimmune disorders are also more common in women.

Estrogen

The sex hormones include estrogens, progesterone, and androgens. Estrogen is the main female sex hormone. It has important effects on female reproductive development, bone health, cardiovascular well-being, and brain function. Estrogen also has important effects on the transmission of pain signals. Progesterone is important for healthy pregnancies. Androgens, such as testosterone, are thought of as male sex hormones, but women also produce androgens that are important for muscle, bone, and skin health, and for maintaining a healthy sex drive. In general, healthy women make less than 10 percent of the amount of testosterone that men do.

THE SEX HORMONES		
Type of Hormone	**Individual Sex Hormones**	**Functions of the Sex Hormones**
Estrogens	Estradiol	Estradiol is the most potent naturally occurring estrogen. It is high in younger women, and levels drop during menopause.
	Estriol	Estriol is the main estrogen produced by the placenta during pregnancy.
	Estrone	Estrone is the main estrogen produced during menopause.
Progesterone	Progesterone	Progesterone helps prepare the uterus for pregnancy and maintains a healthy pregnancy.
Androgens	Dehydroepiandrosterone (DHEA)	DHEA is the main androgen for both men and women. It breaks down to become testosterone and androstenedione.
	Testosterone	Higher testosterone levels in men give them more bone and muscle mass than women.
	Androstenedione	Androstenedione breaks down to become the estrogens estradiol and estrone plus testosterone.

Estradiol affects the communication of pain messages between different parts of the nervous system. Changing levels of estradiol during the menstrual cycle are linked to a cycling of sensitivity to pain.

Some of this is a direct effect of estradiol, and some is because estradiol changes the levels of other brain pain chemicals, including dopamine, endorphins, gamma amino-butyric acid (GABA), norepinephrine, and serotonin. The link between estradiol and pain suggests that women with chronic pain problems might notice changes with menses, pregnancy, and menopause.

Estrogen is also important for digestive symptoms. In an article in the *American Journal of Gastroenterology*, researchers from Hershey Medical Center catalogued many differences between irritable bowel syndrome (IBS) in men and women. Irritable bowel syndrome is more common and problematic for women, and sex hormones such as estrogen may be responsible for differences in digestion between men and women. For example, *gastric motility*—the rate at which food moves through the gastrointestinal tract, including stomach emptying—is slower in women than in men. Estrogen also affects how women experience pain in the digestive organs—called *visceral pain*. These differences also can affect treatment outcome. For example, women experience better relief in controlling diarrhea from IBS when using the drug alosetron (Lotronex®), compared to men.

What to Expect During Your Menstrual Cycle

A variety of painful medical conditions have been reported to worsen with the monthly cycle, including chronic headaches (such as migraines), IBS, and rheumatoid arthritis. A survey of Canadian women with fibromyalgia conducted by researchers at the University of Western Ontario found that most women with fibromyalgia also experience a worsening of their symptoms linked to their menstrual cycles:

▶ Three in four women who were not using any hormone treatment had fibromyalgia symptoms that cycled along with their menstrual cycle, with half of them experiencing a flare just before menstruation.

▶ Four in five women who were using a hormone treatment, such as birth control pills, had fibromyalgia symptoms that cycled with the menses. One in three women on birth control experienced a flare right before her period.

A Norwegian study of women with fibromyalgia also found a worsening of fibromyalgia symptoms before the onset of menses in three out of four women. This survey also asked women with fibromyalgia what

Fibromyalgia symptoms typically flare just before menstruation.

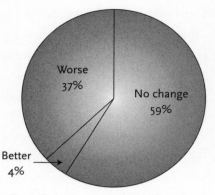

Will taking birth control pills affect my fibromyalgia symptoms?

they experienced when using oral contraceptives. There was no worsening of symptoms for over half of the women taking birth control pills.

What to Expect During Pregnancy

Chapter 10 provides detailed information on how to plan for pregnancy, and the treatments considered safest to use during pregnancy and when nursing. The effect of pregnancy on fibromyalgia was evaluated by comparing 40 pregnancies in women who had fibromyalgia at the time of their pregnancies to 41 pregnancies that occurred in women who experienced fibromyalgia symptoms *only* after they had completed having their children. Having fibromyalgia didn't affect the pregnancies; the women in the study—with and without fibromyalgia—tended to have normal pregnancies and healthy babies.

Having fibromyalgia poses no increased risk of miscarriage or pregnancy complications.

However, fibromyalgia symptoms are likely to worsen during pregnancy and delivery. They tend to be most severe during the third trimester of pregnancy. The most common symptom that women with fibromyalgia have during pregnancy is widespread pain. Fatigue, joint

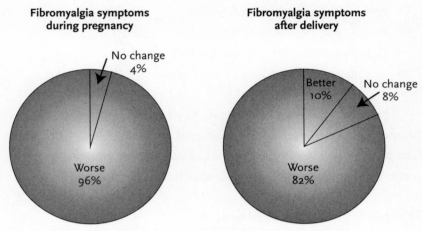

Fibromyalgia symptoms during pregnancy

No change 4%

Worse 96%

Fibromyalgia symptoms after delivery

Better 10%

No change 8%

Worse 82%

What might happen when I'm pregnant, in terms of my fibromyalgia?

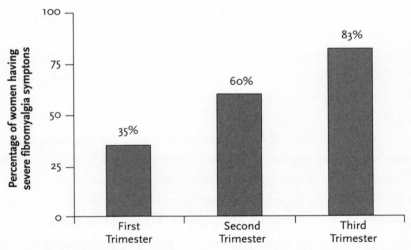

When during pregnancy will my fibromyalgia probably cause the most difficulties?

pain, back pain, depression, weakness, stiffness, and disability can also be issues for women with fibromyalgia during pregnancy.

You may also continue to experience more fibromyalgia symptoms after delivery—fibromyalgia symptoms will be more troublesome for four out of five women:

▶ Pain worsens for three in five women.

▶ Fatigue also worsens for three in five women.

▶ Depression worsens for two in five women.

▶ Anxiety increases for one in five women.

Nursing a baby does not appear to affect fibromyalgia symptoms. In one study, fibromyalgia symptoms did not change with nursing for four in five new mothers. Symptoms improved with nursing for 3 percent of breastfeeding mothers and worsened for 18 percent.

What to Expect With Menopause

The same researchers from the University of Western Ontario also found a link between menopause and fibromyalgia:

▶ One in five women reported that the cyclical changes of fibromyalgia symptoms stopped with menopause.

▶ Taking hormones after menopause affected the symptoms of fibromyalgia for one in three women, with most of them reporting a benefit from taking hormones.

A possible effect of hormone replacement on fibromyalgia symptoms was further explored in an important study published in 2011, in the journal *Rheumatology*. Postmenopausal women with fibromyalgia were randomly assigned to receive an estrogen patch as a hormone replacement for 8 weeks or a *placebo*, an identical-looking patch that didn't contain medication. The women were asked about their pain and tested for pain sensitivity using cold, heat, and pressure before they started the patch, after wearing the patch for 2 months, and 5 months after they had stopped using it. There were generally no important pain differences between using the patch or not, or between women using the hormone patch compared with the placebo. This indicates that women with fibromyalgia who need to use hormone therapy for menopause should not expect to experience any changes in overall pain symptoms, pain threshold, or pain tolerance.

Hormone therapy is often used during early menopause for issues such as hot flashes, mood swings, and vaginal dryness. The Endocrine Society developed recommendations for its safe use in 2010:

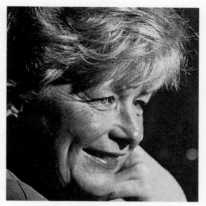

▶ Hormone replacement therapy is best used when treating younger women (especially women under 60).

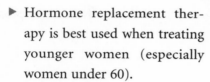
Taking hormone replacement after menopause is not expected to change fibromyalgia symptoms for better or worse.

▶ It can be used to treat early menopause symptoms.
▶ Hormone replacement therapy should generally last no more than 5 years.

Hormone replacement may have the additional benefits of preventing fractures and the development of diabetes. Always talk to your doctor before starting any hormone therapy to make sure you are a good candidate for this treatment.

SUMMARY

▶ Many different abnormalities are present in people with fibromyalgia, although we're not sure which ones may be the cause of fibromyalgia.
▶ People with fibromyalgia are more sensitive to pain because of changes in the brain and nervous system.
▶ Microscopic changes in type II muscle fibers may result in weakness and fatigue.

▶ Fibromyalgia runs in families, and researchers are beginning to identify genes that may be linked to an increased risk for developing it.

▶ Important hormonal factors that affect fibromyalgia may include reduced effects from growth hormone and the presence of thyroid antibodies.

▶ Fibromyalgia symptoms may cycle with changing estrogen levels. Symptoms are often aggravated with menses and during the later stages of pregnancy.

▶ Taking hormone replacement therapy to treat the early troublesome symptoms of menopause is unlikely to affect fibromyalgia pain levels.

Part III

Fibromyalgia Treatments That Really Work

Managing your fibromyalgia will probably involve several types of treatment, rather than a single modality, because symptoms are usually complicated and diverse.

It will take a few weeks before you'll start to notice improvement with a new therapy. Use the tools in Chapter 11 to track your progress, so you can see what treatment or combination of treatments is most helpful for you. It's important to remember that no one treatment is likely to result in a dramatic reduction in symptoms. Often, you won't see the "light at the end of the tunnel" until you are using several treatments, each adding a bit of improvement. As you read through this section, you'll notice that most treatments help reduce pain, but not every treatment works well for other symptoms, including poor sleep, fatigue, and mood disturbance. Make sure you target your most difficult symptoms. Irritable bowel syndrome (IBS) or migraine may also need additional individualized treatments.

Everyone with fibromyalgia is different. Exercise and behavioral therapies help most people with fibromyalgia, and a variety of medications and nutritional supplements may be useful, but you will probably need to try various treatments to determine which combination is helpful for you.

Non-drug treatments are among the most effective therapies for fibromyalgia, and often several are combined—you might find that you get the best results by using two or three non-drug therapies, or possibly a combination of several non-drug treatments, a prescription medication, and a nutritional supplement.

Non-drug therapies don't involve taking medication; they change the physiology of brain chemicals and target the muscles, joints, and soft tissues. The changes in brain chemicals produced by using non-drug methods such as relaxation techniques are the same type of changes that you might achieve by taking pain-relieving drugs. The most obvious advantage is that you don't have to worry about medication side effects.

Non-drug treatments can be divided into two categories:

1. Physical treatments such as aerobic exercise, and
2. Behavioral treatments such as cognitive-behavioral therapy.

Psychologists often teach behavioral strategies. These methods do not address underlying emotional problems in fibromyalgia—rather, they involve specific techniques that relieve pain. Physical therapists, occupational therapists, and nurses may also teach behavioral treatments and relaxation techniques.

The number of effective medications for fibromyalgia is limited. If your doctor doesn't prescribe pain medications (analgesics) for your painful fibromyalgia, it's not because he doesn't believe your pain is real. For reasons we don't entirely understand, pain medications only help relieve certain types of pain and are generally not very helpful for fibromyalgia.

Some prescription and nutritional therapies can help reduce a range of fibromyalgia symptoms, but no drugs have been developed specifically for fibromyalgia. Instead, drugs that were originally designed to treat mood disorders or other nervous system diseases have been found to also correct chemical imbalances in fibromyalgia and reduce symptoms.

Finally, women with fibromyalgia are often concerned about what treatments are safe while trying to get pregnant, during pregnancy, after the baby is born, and while breastfeeding. It's important to know whether it's safe to use the same treatment(s) that were used before pregnancy, and what other therapies might be especially helpful in targeting symptoms during pregnancy.

Fibromyalgia treatment is not simple. You probably won't find that simply doing yoga or taking a certain pill will be all you need. The *good* news is that the broad range of available treatments is effective for many people. Having a closet full of treatments that you can pull out and use on different days will help keep your fibromyalgia symptoms in check and reduce your disability.

6

Exercise and Other Physical Treatments

When you're sore and achy all over, the last thing you might want to do is exercise. Years ago, doctors usually prescribed rest—even strict bed rest—for patients with severe pain, because they believed that resting painful muscles and joints would help make the pain go away faster. Since then, we've learned that our bodies are designed to *move* and that pain can actually worsen when we don't exercise.

For example, although early astronauts were in top physical condition when they went on space missions, two in three developed moderate or severe back pain while in space. This occurred because they were floating in space without gravity and didn't believe they needed to exercise. Now, astronauts work out on treadmills or do other types of exercise while on missions. Lack of exercise, even in space, worsens pain.

Your fibromyalgia didn't start because of lack of exercise, but exercising can be an important tool in reducing the pain messages coming from your muscles and joints. A review by researchers from the University of Saskatchewan of nearly 50 exercise programs resulted in specific recommendations for people with fibromyalgia that include combining aerobic exercise and strength training. Alternating a day of aerobic exercise with a day of strength training can be a good way to achieve these exercise targets.

EXERCISE RECOMMENDATIONS FOR FIBROMYALGIA

Type of Exercise	Daily Exercise Requirement	Recommended Frequency
Aerobic exercise gradually increased to moderate intensity	At least 20 minutes total, which can be divided into two 10-minute sessions	2–3 days per week
Strength training	8–12 repetitions per exercise	2–3 days per week

Exercise reduces pain, increases physical fitness and overall well-being, and improves mood. Although it may not improve poor sleep, researchers from the University of North Carolina showed that aerobic exercise also reduces fatigue and "fibro fog." In this study, 16 women with fibromyalgia were randomly assigned to either an 18-week exercise program or a control group that was monitored but not treated. The exercise included walking, light resistance exercise, and stretching for 60 minutes, 3 days per week. Women assigned to the exercise group completed about two-thirds of the exercise sessions. Following treatment, they felt mentally sharper and performed better on memory recall tests.

If you also have chronic fatigue syndrome, you may find that your fibromyalgia symptoms worsen after exercise. Make sure you start slowly, and increase your exercise intensity gradually to avoid increasing your symptoms.

The benefits of exercise usually don't happen right away. In many cases, exercise needs to be performed consistently for 4–6 weeks before you begin to experience benefits. You *will* need to continue your exercise program to experience long-lasting benefits.

EXERCISES THAT HELP FIBROMYALGIA

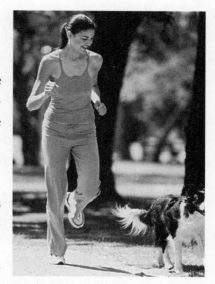

Exercise has proved to be one of the most helpful treatments for reducing fibromyalgia symptoms. The most effective exercises include:

- ▶ Aerobic exercise:
  - Do whole-body stretches before beginning your workout.
  - After a 5-minute warm-up, exercise for a total of 20 minutes, followed by a 5-minute cool-down.

Aerobic exercise improves pain, mood, fatigue, and fibro fog.

  - Do aerobic exercise at least 4 days per week.
  - Doing aerobic exercise in warm water may be beneficial.
- ▶ Strength training:
  - Work up to doing 8–12 repetitions per strength exercise.
  - Do strength training 2–3 days per week.

Fibromyalgia expert Dr. Winfried Häuser reviewed studies regarding the effects of aerobic exercise as a treatment for fibromyalgia. Here's a summary of the findings published in *Arthritis Research & Therapy*:

- ▶ Aerobic exercise, including water aerobics, helps reduce fibromyalgia symptoms.
- ▶ There is no difference in benefits if you do aerobic exercise on land or in water.
- ▶ In addition to improving physical fitness in people with fibromyalgia, aerobic exercise significantly decreases pain, fatigue, and depressed mood.

▶ Start aerobics at a comfortable level and gradually increase to a target of low- to moderate-intensity exercise for 20–30 minutes, 2–3 times a week. At moderate intensity, you should be able to have a conversation with someone while you exercise.

▶ Stick with your aerobic program for at least 4–6 weeks to see benefits.

▶ People who continue an exercise program are more likely to have less pain and depression than those who stop.

Dr. Häuser cautions that people with fibromyalgia might experience a minimal increase in pain and fatigue when they first start a new exercise program. Any increase should be tolerable and improve over the first few weeks. If your symptoms become more extreme or persistent, talk to your doctor or exercise trainer about modifying your program.

Keeping track of your exercise progress in a daily diary can help motivate you to stick with your program. You will find exercise logs in Chapter 11. Share these logs with your health care provider to help assess your program and its benefits.

Talk to your doctor before starting any exercise program to help determine what's best for you. Among the many possibilities, good aerobic exercise might include biking, swimming, or walking in the mall, on hiking trails, or on a school track.

Developing Your Exercise Program

Start your aerobics program at a level that's comfortable for you in intensity and duration. Gradually work up to:

▶ Moderate-intensity exercise (You should be able to talk but not sing while exercising.)

▶ 20–30 minutes per exercise session

▶ Three days a week—preferably alternating days doing aerobic exercise and strength training

Setting Your Pace

When you start a new aerobic exercise program, work gradually toward your goal. Physiotherapy experts from the University College Antwerp have suggested the following strategy to find your target:

1. First, determine how long you can comfortably exercise without an increase in symptoms. This is your "comfort time."

2. When you're having a good day:
   - Exercise for 75 percent of your comfort time.
   - Rest for 75 percent of your comfort time.
   - Exercise for 75 percent of your comfort time.

3. When you're having a bad day:
   - Exercise for 50 percent of your comfort time.
   - Rest for 50 percent of your comfort time.
   - Exercise for 50 percent of your comfort time.

Here's an example:

▶ You are walking for your aerobic exercise, and your comfort time is 20 minutes.

▶ On days when you're feeling good, walk for 15 minutes, rest for 15 minutes, and then do another 15-minute walk.

▶ On days when you're having symptom flares, walk for 10 minutes, rest for 10 minutes, and walk for another 10 minutes.

Begin any new aerobic program slowly, and increase the intensity every 4–5 days. If your pain worsens, temporarily reduce your activity to the level that you previously tolerated for 2–3 days, then try increasing it again.

Make Your Exercise Program a Success

Ask any physician what the best treatment is for fibromyalgia, and she will probably tell you *Exercise!* Although research consistently shows the benefits of aerobic exercise, most people with fibromyalgia don't exercise. Researchers from the Oregon Health & Science University recently reported that four in five people with fibromyalgia do *no* aerobic exercise. An increase in soreness and fatigue was the most common reason given for not exercising.

If people know that exercise is helpful for fibromyalgia but still don't do it, what's the problem? It's definitely not because they don't want to get better. It's more likely because exercise is more difficult when you have fibromyalgia, for several reasons:

▶ During exercise, blood flow increases to muscles to bring important nutrients and remove wastes from the tissues. If wastes, such as lactic acid, build up in the muscles, anyone can develop exercise-related pain. Blood flow to the muscles during exercise is lower than normal in people with fibromyalgia, making exercise more painful.

▶ Normally, exercise helps reduce pain by increasing pain-blocking brain chemicals, such as endorphins. However, these pain-blocking pathways are less active and less responsive in people with fibromyalgia, which is another reason why exercise may be more painful.

▶ People with fibromyalgia have reduced exercise tolerance. They may have abnormalities in the autonomic nervous system, which controls heart rate and blood pressure, and this, in turn, increases fatigue.

▶ Hormonal factors may also play a role. For example, growth hormone helps repair the tiny muscle tears (*muscle microtrauma*) that occur with exercise. The deficiencies in growth hormone associated with fibromyalgia may impair this repair mechanism.

Despite this, it's important to develop a consistent exercise program when you have fibromyalgia. Choose a type of exercise that is the most compatible with your physical limitations, lifestyle, and interests. In general, walking is one of the best exercises—you get a great workout, you don't need special equipment, and it's free. But if you're not interested in walking, biking, or swimming, most fibromyalgia studies show that a wide range of other exercises can be helpful. For example, a study from the University of Uludag in Turkey recently reported benefits from Pilates training.

Choose an exercise you tolerate and enjoy, and that doesn't cause excessive pain flares. As you become more comfortable with exercising, increase your exercise duration and intensity.

Tips for Making Exercise a Success

▶ *Start low and go slow.* Choose an exercise you think you will enjoy and start at a level that's comfortable for you. Exercise at this level for at least 1 week before trying to increase your exercise duration or intensity. Alternate increasing duration and intensity—don't increase both together—and then stay with one level without increasing the other until you've been comfortable during exercise for at least 1 week.

▶ *Choose an appropriate intensity level.* You should be able to chat with someone when you're exercising, but not sing. If you can sing, you're not working hard enough. If you can't talk comfortably, slow down.

▶ *Don't forget to stretch before and after aerobic exercise.* In general, stretching exercises are less helpful for people with fibromyalgia than for people with other types of chronic pain. But don't completely forego stretching; it's essential to help your muscles get warm, flexible, and ready for exercise—and to cool down after exercise. Stretching also helps reduce your risk for injury and pain flares.

▶ *Plan your exercise for the time of day when your fatigue is usually the least.* If you typically take a short nap in the afternoon, try exercising after your nap, when you feel rested.

▶ *Make exercise part of your daily routine.* Don't decide on a day-by-day basis if you should exercise that day—make it a must-do, as with brushing your

(continued on next page)

teeth or styling your hair. If you're having a particularly bad day, cut back on exercise rather than cutting it out. Once you start missing here and there, it's easy to stop exercising altogether. Scheduling daily walks or doing your exercise in front of your favorite daily television shows can encourage you to find time for exercise.

▶ *Find a reliable exercise buddy.* Having an exercise partner is one of the most powerful motivators for sticking with an exercise program. Select someone whose physical abilities are similar to yours, so you don't go too fast or too slow. A great walking buddy—and one who never accepts an excuse for skipping a day of exercise—might be your dog!

▶ *Measure your exercise duration in minutes, not distance.* Measuring time is easier.

▶ *Get a new pair of exercise shoes at least every 6 months.* Exercising in old shoes can increase pain and the risk for injury.

▶ *If you have problems with stiff joints,* try exercising in a warm swimming pool rather than an air-conditioned gym.

SPECIFIC EXERCISES FOR PEOPLE WITH FIBROMYALGIA

Whole-Body Stretches

Begin and end each exercise session with 10–15 minutes of stretching. These exercises are an important way to help prepare your muscles and joints for aerobic exercise. They can also help you wind down at the end of the day before going to bed. You may want to try these stretches after taking a warm shower. If your muscles are sore when you finish stretching, put a heating pad or a cool pack—whichever you find most soothing—over the sorest areas for 10 minutes.

Perform each stretch *slowly*. Stretch until you first feel the stretching sensation. Then hold the stretch for 5 seconds, relax, and repeat 3–10 times. Try doing the specific stretches given in this chapter while you listen to music. If your pain levels consistently increase after stretching, reduce the extent of the stretches and review your exercise program with your physical therapist.

Starting Position for Stretching

Lie flat on the floor. If you feel uncomfortable lying on your back, bend your knees and press the small of your back into the floor.

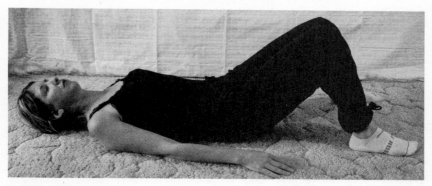

Neck Rotation

Start by looking up at the ceiling. Then rotate your neck slowly to the left. Try to place your left ear flat on the floor. Hold for 5 seconds. Return to center and relax. Then rotate to the right and hold for 5 seconds. Return to center and relax.

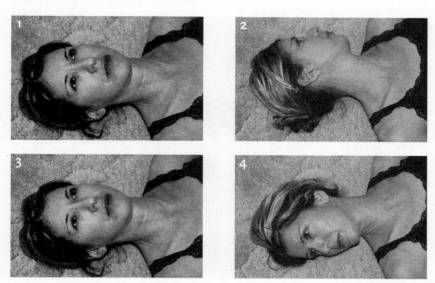

Shoulder Rollover

Hold each arm out at the shoulder, so your body makes a giant cross. Keeping your arms flat on the floor, bend your elbows to make a 90-degree angle. This is your starting position. Keep your arms on the floor between the shoulder and elbow, and rotate your forearms up and over. Then rotate back to the starting position.

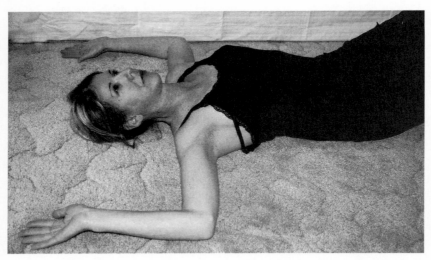

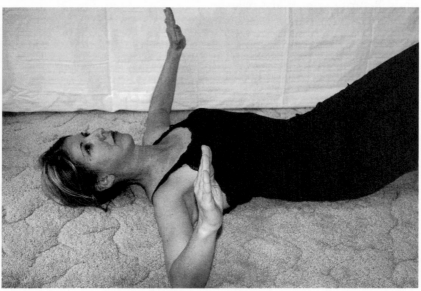

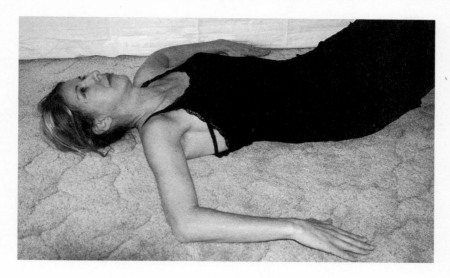

Shoulder Stick 'Em Up

Take a deep breath and raise your arms over your head, as if someone just said, "Stick 'em up!" Breathe out and reach around with your arms in a half circle, first up toward the ceiling, then down to your sides. Breathe in and reach overhead again.

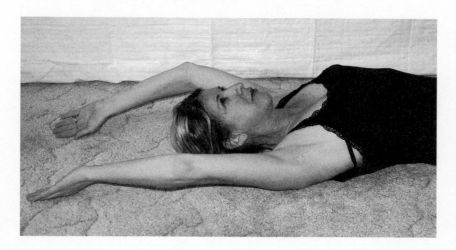

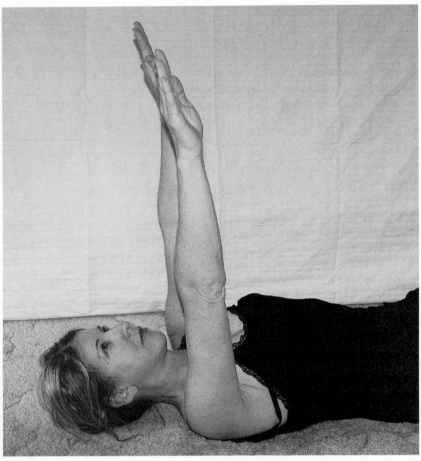

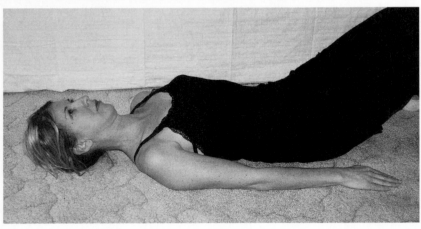

Upper Body Twist

Lift your left arm toward the ceiling and grab your left wrist with your right hand. Keeping your left arm straight (don't bend your left elbow), pull your left arm across your chest to the right. Then turn your chin to the left. Hold. Repeat with the right arm.

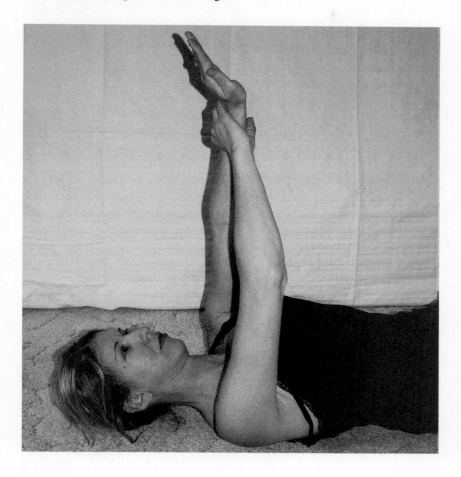

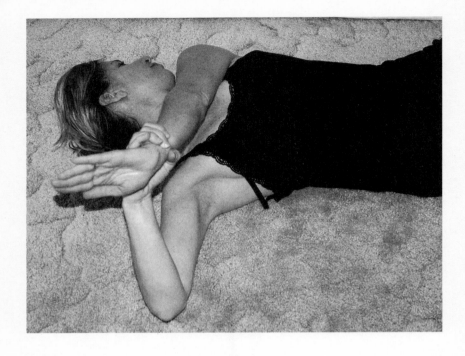

Reach Away

Stretch your left arm over your head and point your right toe. Stretch your arm and leg away from each other. Hold. Repeat with the right arm and left leg.

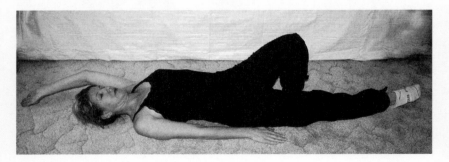

Knee to Chest

Lie on your back. Pull one knee toward your chest and hold for 5–8 seconds. Feel the gentle pulling sensation in your buttock. Return your leg to straight position. Repeat five times. Repeat with the other leg.

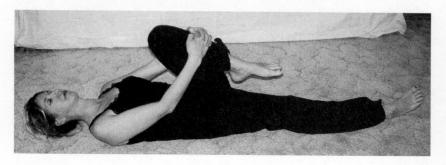

Pelvic Twist

Make sure you begin this stretch with your knees bent and the small of your back pressed into the floor. Throughout this stretch, keep your knees together and your shoulders touching the floor. Slowly lower your knees toward the floor to the right, causing your pelvis to rotate. Turn your head to the left, away from your knees. Hold. Return knees and head to the center. Then lower your knees to the left and look to the right. Keep your head and shoulders on the floor to allow your pelvis to rotate.

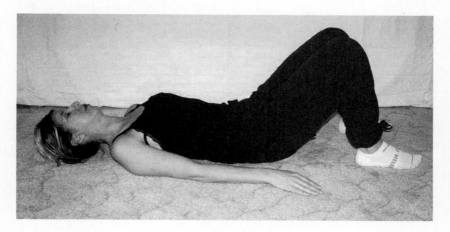

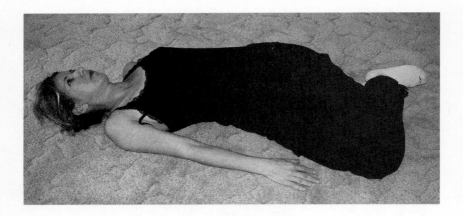

Hip Stretch

Begin this stretch with your knees bent and the small of your back pressed into the floor. Throughout this stretch, keep your shoulders touching the floor. Bend your left leg and put your ankle on your right knee. Gently press against your left knee, feeling the stretch in your hip and upper leg. Repeat with your other leg.

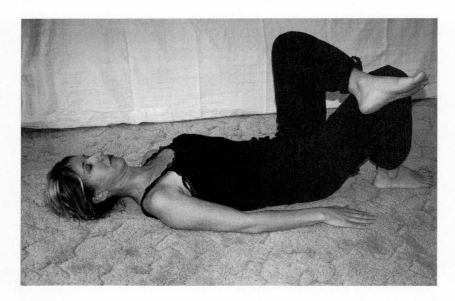

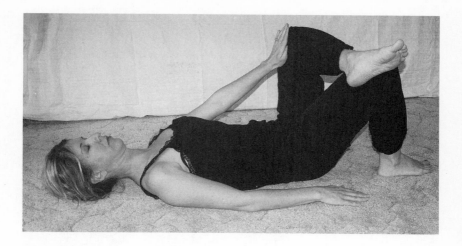

Happy Feet

Spread your feet about 2 feet apart. Turn the toes together in the middle. Hold. Then turn both feet so your toes are far away from each other. Hold. Point toes away from you. Hold. Then pull toes up toward you. Hold.

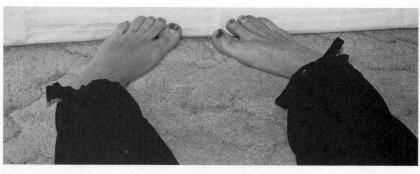

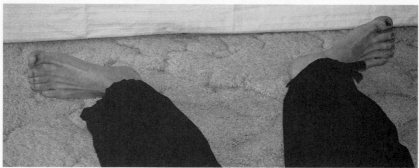

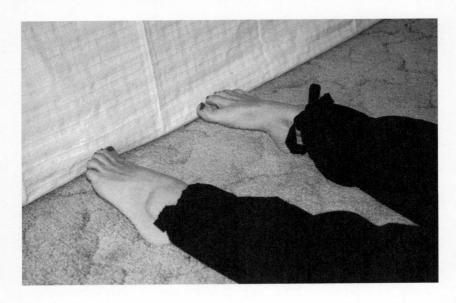

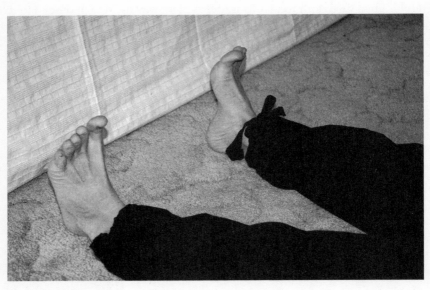

Calf Stretch

Stand behind a sturdy chair, holding onto the back of the chair. Move your right foot back 2–3 feet and keep your feet flat on the ground. Bend your left knee. You will feel a stretch in the back of your right leg and calf. Hold. Repeat with the other leg.

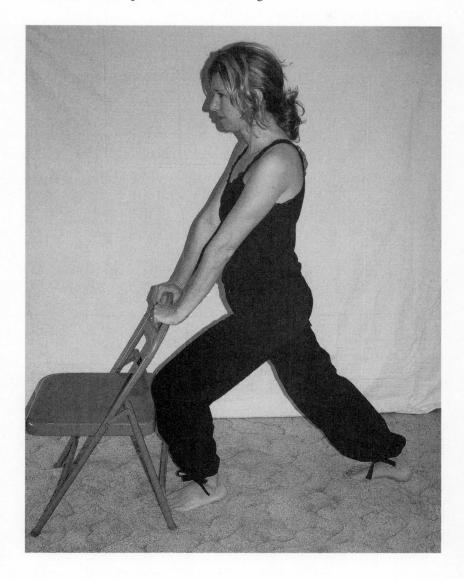

Strength Exercises

Toe Lift

Stand behind a sturdy chair, holding onto the back of the chair. Lift up your body so you are standing on your toes. Hold for 5–8 seconds. Lower your heels to the floor. Repeat five times.

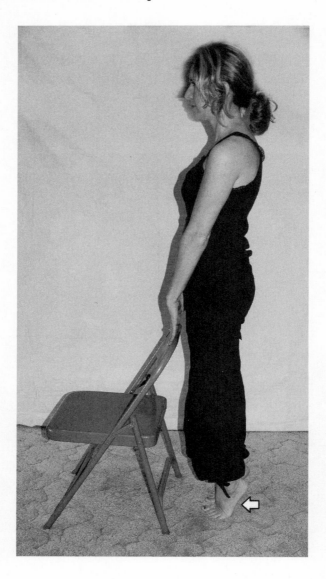

Hip and Thigh Builders

Stand behind a sturdy chair, holding onto the back of the chair. Bend your left leg and hold for 5 seconds. Repeat 5–10 times. Repeat with other leg.

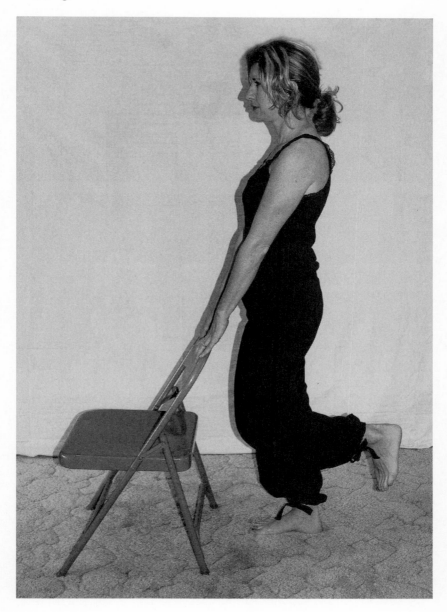

Turn 90 degrees and hold onto the back of the chair for support. Lift your left knee and hold for 5 seconds. Repeat 5–10 times. Repeat with other leg. Then lift your left leg out to the side and hold for 5 seconds. Repeat 5–10 times. Repeat with other leg.

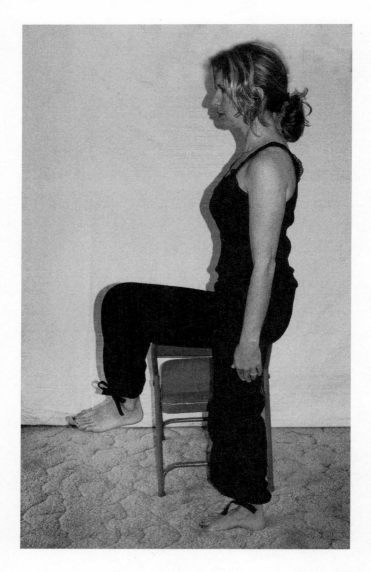

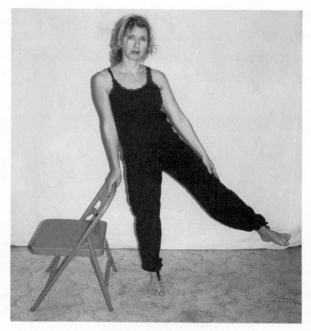

Sit in the chair with your back against the back of the chair and feet flat on the floor. Straighten one leg and hold for 5 seconds. Repeat 5–10 times. Repeat with other leg.

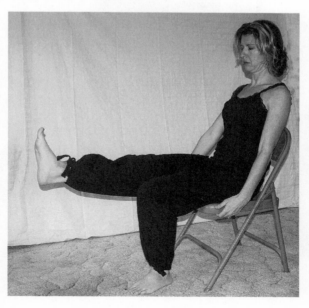

Arm Builders

Sit in a chair with your back against the back of the chair and feet flat on the floor. Hang your arms at your sides. Lift your arms out to the side and hold for 5–10 seconds.

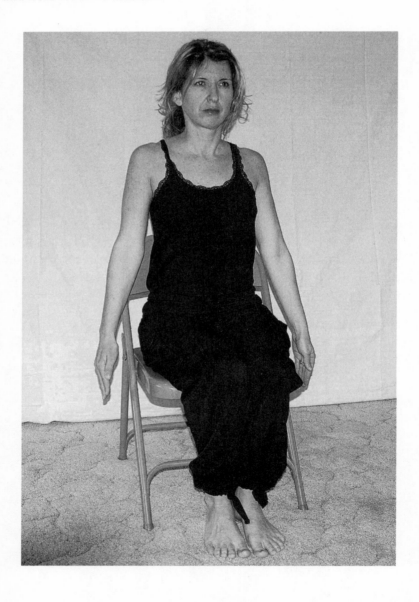

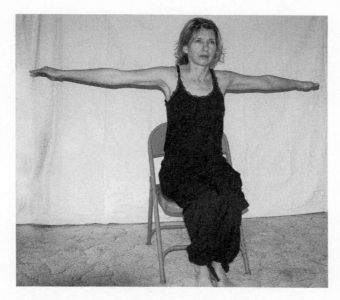

Return your arms to your sides and turn them so your palms are facing forward. Then lift your arms in front of you, with your palms facing the ceiling. Hold 5–10 seconds.

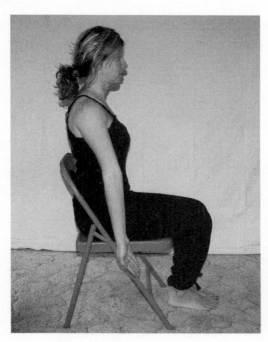

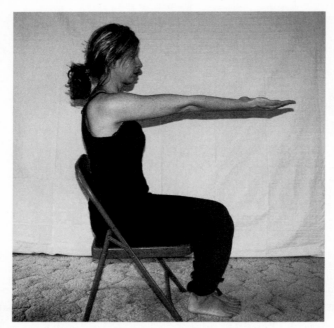

Lower your arms to your sides and turn your palms so they face toward your body. Then raise your arms in front of you with your palms facing the floor. Hold 5–10 seconds.

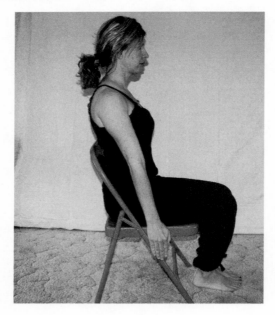

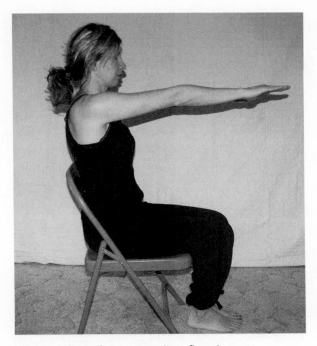

Repeat this series of arm exercises five times.

Isometrics

Sit in a chair with your back against the back of the chair and feet flat on the floor. Bend your elbow and place your left fist in your right hand above your lap. Push down with your fist at the same time you are pushing up with your palm. Your hands should stay in the same position without moving. Push for 5–10 seconds. Then relax and repeat five times.

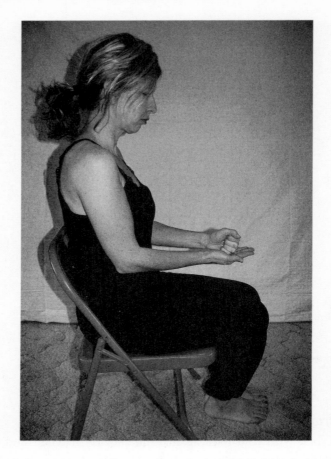

Bend your elbows and interlace your fingers in front of your chest. Try to pull your elbows apart, keeping your fingers interlocked. Pull for 5–10 seconds. Then relax and repeat five times.

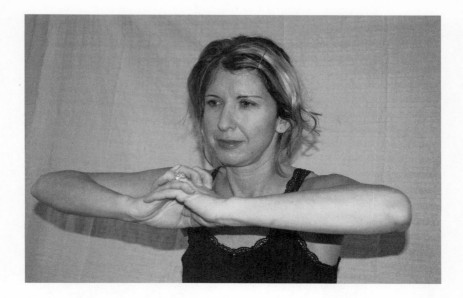

Bend your elbows and press your fists against each other in front of your chest. Push for 5–10 seconds. Then relax and repeat five times.

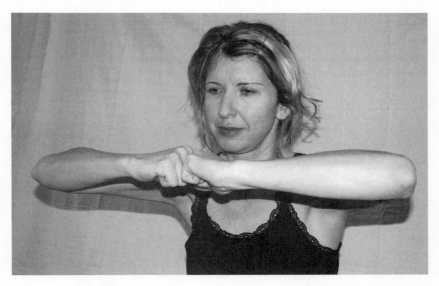

Place your palm against the front of your head. Press your head forward and hand backward. Your head should not move. Push for 5–10 seconds. Then relax and repeat five times. Next, press your hand against the left side of the head, while pushing back with your head to keep your head from moving. Push for 5–10 seconds. Then relax and repeat five times. Repeat on the other side of your head.

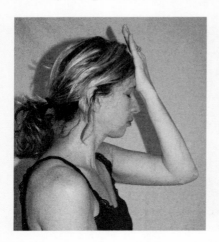 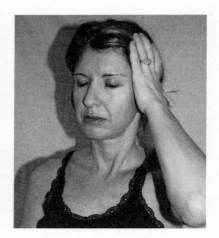

Put both hands behind your head. Press your head forward with your hands while pushing your head backward. Your head should not move. Push for 5–10 seconds. Then relax and repeat five times.

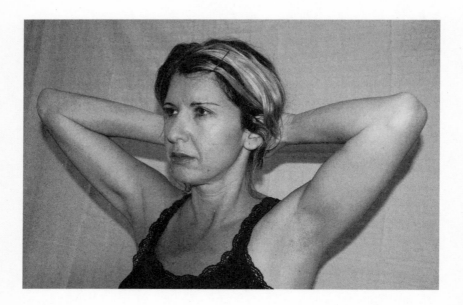

Push-Ups

Stand behind a sturdy chair, holding onto the back of the chair. Your arms should be about shoulder-width apart. Step back about 4–5 feet from the chair. Bend your arms and keep your back straight so that your chest moves toward the chair. Don't bend your arms more than 90 degrees. Then straighten your arms to return to the starting position. Repeat 5–10 times.

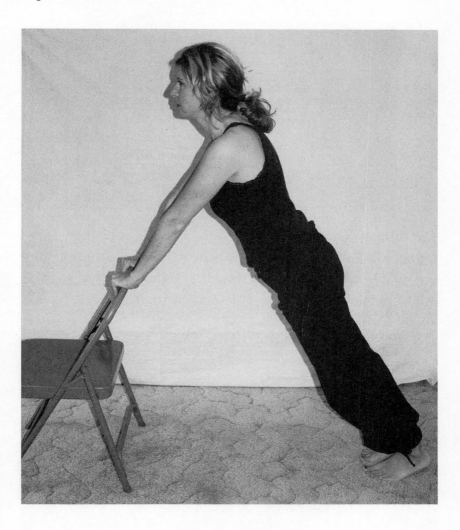

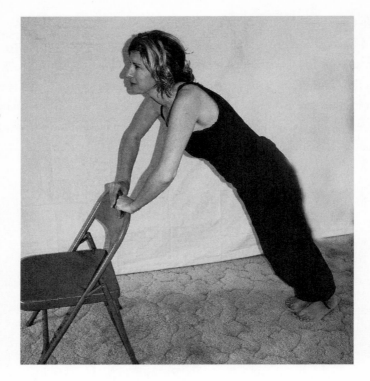

Gut Buster

Lie on your back with your knees bent and the small of your back pressed into the floor. Lift your shoulders off the floor while grabbing behind your knees. Hold for 5–10 seconds. Relax. Repeat 5–10 times.

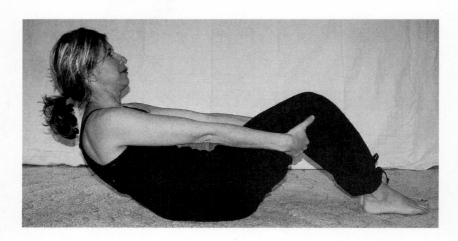

Water Therapy

Therapeutic hydrotherapy may include balneotherapy (drinking or bathing in medicinal water), bathing in warm or cold water or mud, and spa therapy (drinking or bathing in thermal or mineral waters). A review of ten well-designed research studies testing the effects of hydrotherapy in a total of 446 people with fibromyalgia showed significant reductions in pain and improvements in quality of life. The largest individual study randomly assigned 80 people who were being treated with medication to either continue their usual medications, or take their usual medications plus have 12 mud packs and 12 thermal baths administered over 2 weeks.

There was no change in pain or disability in the people who merely continued their usual medications when they were retested 2 weeks and 16 weeks later. In contrast, the group that also used hydrotherapy had a 19 percent reduction in pain and a 23 percent drop in disability after 2 weeks. These benefits were not just short-term; reductions in pain and disability were still seen 14 weeks after completing therapy.

Another beneficial type of water therapy is aquatic therapy, which involves performing exercises in warm pool water. Performing exercises in warm water provides soothing benefits, and the water's buoyancy provides added support. People who have arthritis or joint stiffness in addition to fibromyalgia often particularly benefit from doing exercise in warm pool water. "Warm" is usually defined as 90–91°F, or 32–33°C.

Yoga

Yoga is a terrific exercise for fibromyalgia because it combines both strength and balance training. Yoga can reduce pain by relieving muscle tightness, inducing relaxation, and reducing stress. It has fairly consistently shown both short- and long-term benefits for reducing a wide range of fibromyalgia symptoms. Researchers from the Oregon Health

& Science University randomly assigned 53 women with fibromyalgia—who had been using a stable treatment regimen of drug and/or non-drug treatment for at least 3 months—to continue their standard fibromyalgia treatment program or to add eight weekly yoga classes to their treatment. The yoga classes included instruction in meditation, breathing exercises, coping skills, and gentle stretching poses. Participants were advised to practice at home between classes for 20–40 minutes a day.

In the yoga group, pain, fatigue, and poor sleep were reduced by 20–25 percent; mood was improved by 39 percent; and poor memory was reduced by 22 percent. In the group continuing the standard treatment, each symptom was slightly worse at the end of the study period, except that depression was reduced by 11 percent. This study teaches us two important things about fibromyalgia. First, yoga can be a helpful addition to your fibromyalgia treatment routine. Second, when you've been using the same treatments for 3 months or more, you probably won't notice substantial additional benefits from continuing the same treatments. So, if your treatment is helpful, keep it up. But if you've been on a stable treatment program for over 3 months and it's not helping, it might be time to try something else, such as yoga.

There are many different types of yoga, ranging from "restorative" to the more physical "power" yoga. Some people find heated yoga classes healing and therapeutic, while others might find the heat overwhelming. Explore different yoga options to find the style that's best for you. Work with a yoga instructor who can understand any physical limitations you may have and help you develop modifications for those poses that may not be suitable for your body.

Key Guiding Principles in the Practice of Yoga

▶ *Breathing.* Yogic breath is the single most important element of yoga practice. Relax your breathing by breathing in and out slowly through your nose. *Be sure to breathe through your nose and not your mouth.* Controlled breathing helps you link your mind and body, helps you stay focused, and reduces stress.

▶ *Alignment.* Yoga poses need to be performed with your joints properly aligned. The body can be compared to the wheels of a car that wear unevenly when the car is out of alignment. Make sure your joints are aligned while practicing yoga to ensure that your body is stable.

▶ *Drishti.* Drishti is a fixed, relaxed gaze that is practiced in conjunction with yoga. Focus on looking at one spot while in a pose to assist you in staying focused on the pose and to calm your mind.

▶ *Uddiyana Bandha.* Many bandhas, or "locks," are practiced in yoga, but uddiyana bandha is especially important for people suffering from lower back issues. This a core stabilization practiced in every pose. To use uddiyana bandha, draw your abdominal muscles in and up to support your lower spine. This will strengthen and tone your body's core and protect your lower back.

▶ *Respecting/Honoring the Body.* Yoga is the art of listening—most importantly, listening to your body. There are options for modifying any pose. Use modifications any time you feel pain from a pose. The breath is a great tool to gauge your effort level in yoga practice. If you're gasping or struggling for breath, you should either ease up on the pose or stop and rest. Ultimately, yoga practice should make you feel good, so be sure all the poses you use are moving you toward feeling better.

A Simple Yoga Sequence

Yoga instructor Melissa Watts has provided a simple yoga sequence you can use to start exploring the benefits of yoga. This routine includes warm-up, balancing poses, and floor poses.

The Warm-Ups

Child's Pose: This pose awakens the connection between your breath and your body. It is also a resting pose that you can use whenever you need it during your yoga practice.

Get on your hands and knees on your mat. Then bring your big toes together and widen your knees to the edges of your mat. Sink your hips back onto your heels, and rest your forehead onto the mat. Stretch your arms in front of you. Hold for 5–10 breaths, or until you feel ready to begin doing yoga.

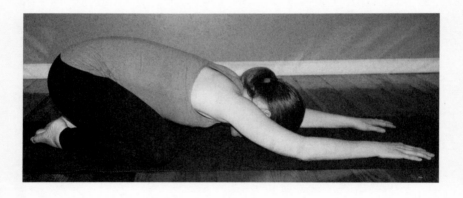

Cat and Cow: This pose gently stretches and awakens the spine.

From Child's Pose, come onto your hands and knees. Align your wrists under your shoulders, and align your knees under your hips. Inhale and lift your chest and tailbone to make the Cow Pose.

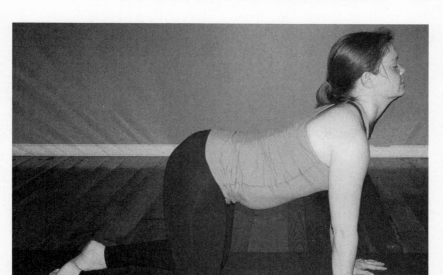

Then exhale, drop your head, and round your back to make the Cat Pose.

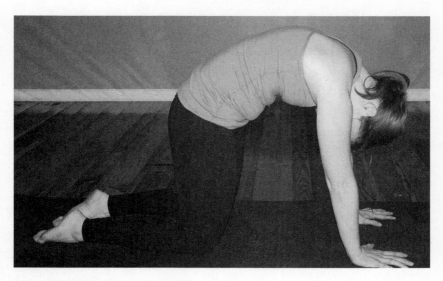

Repeat for five or more breaths.

Downward Facing Dog: This pose awakens the whole body. It lengthens your spine as you lift up through your tailbone, builds shoulder and arm strength, and provides calming.

From Cat/Cow pose, walk your hands forward while keeping them shoulder-width apart. Press into your palms, curl your toes under, and lift your hips up toward the ceiling. Your feet should be hip-width apart, and your gaze should fall between your feet. Be mindful to push forward through your hands, while pressing back through your thighs to keep the weight of the body lifting up through the hips.

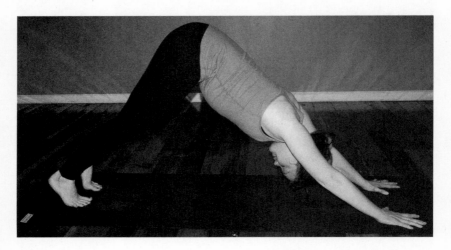

Sun Salutation A: This series of poses links breath and movement together, and starts to engage, strengthen, and stretch all areas of the body.

From Downward Facing Dog, step to the front of your mat. With your feet hip-width apart, fold forward. Now you are in Ragdoll Pose. Take a few breaths and allow the weight of your upper body to relax and lengthen the neck and spine.

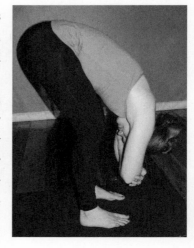

Bring your feet together and roll up to standing. Then inhale as you reach your arms up to the sky.

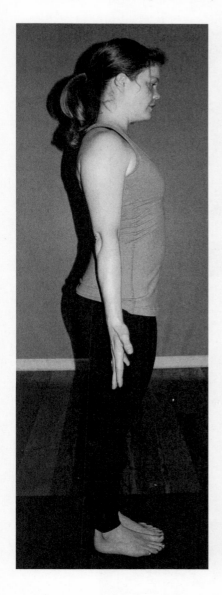
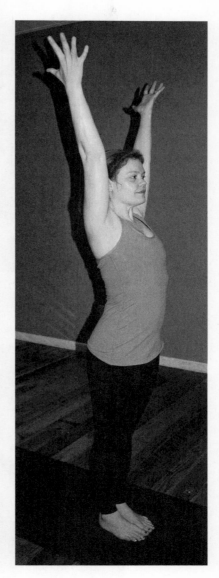

Exhale and fold forward toward the floor.

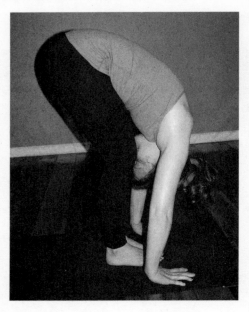

Inhale and lift your chest up to hip height, placing your hands on your knees.

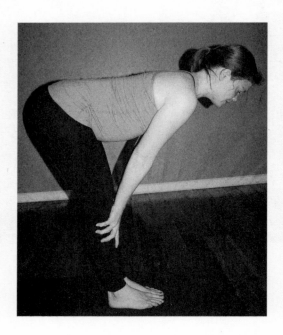

Exhale and step back to a Push-up position. Then drop your knees to the floor.

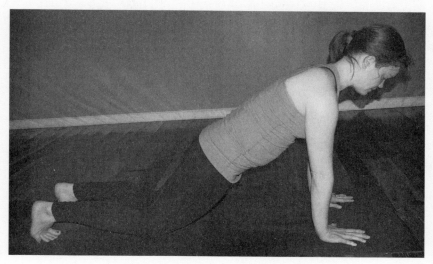

Finally, lower your body all the way to the floor.

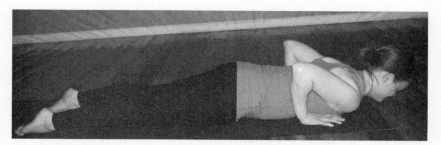

Inhale and lift up your chest to come into Cobra pose.

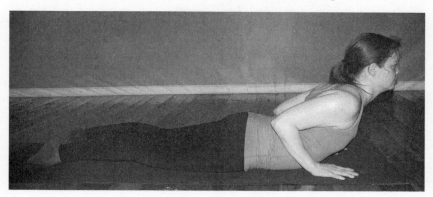

Finally, exhale back to Downward Facing Dog.

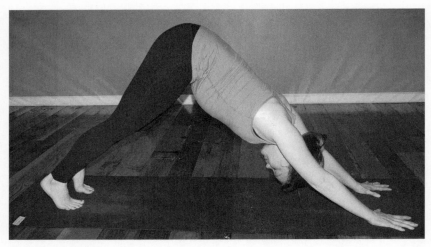

Repeat twice.

Sun Salutation B: This series of poses will help you continue warming up your body with specific emphasis on stretching and strengthening the hips and legs.

Starting from Downward Facing Dog, step forward, and bring your toes and knees together while folding to the floor. Inhale and lift your chest up to hip height. Exhale and fold back to the floor.

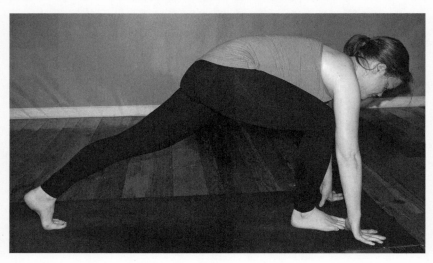

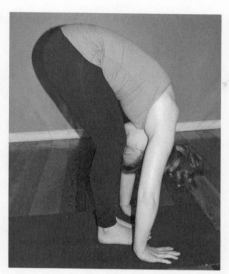

Bend your knees, inhale, and reach your arms to sky to make Thunderbolt Pose.

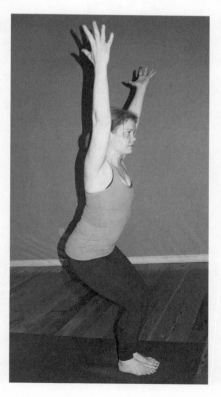

Exhale and fold forward, inhale to halfway lift, and exhale to Push-up position.

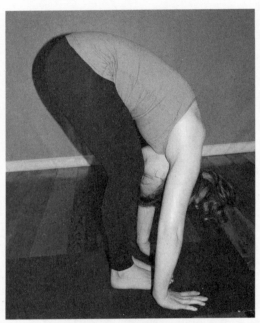

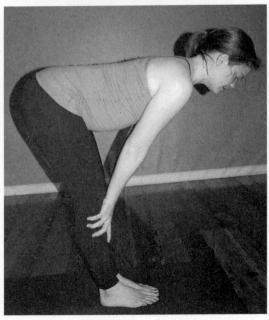

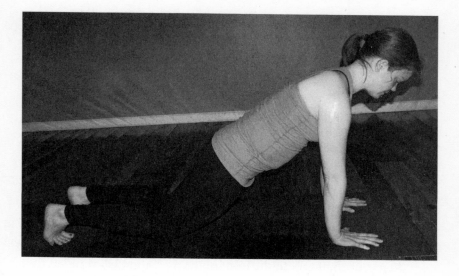

Lower to the floor as you continue to exhale. Then inhale to Cobra pose. Finally, exhale back to Downward Facing Dog.

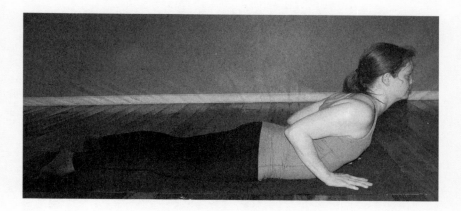

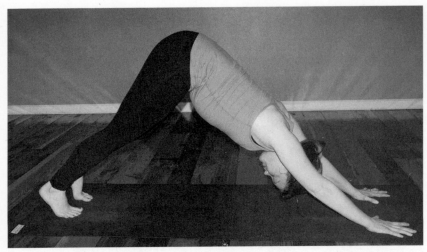

Step your right foot to the front of the mat, and turn your left foot flat for the Warrior 1 pose.

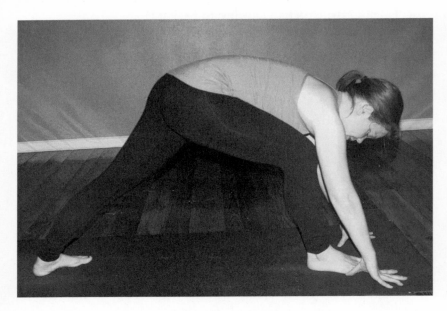

Push into your feet as you reach up through your arms, trying to square hips to the front of the room.

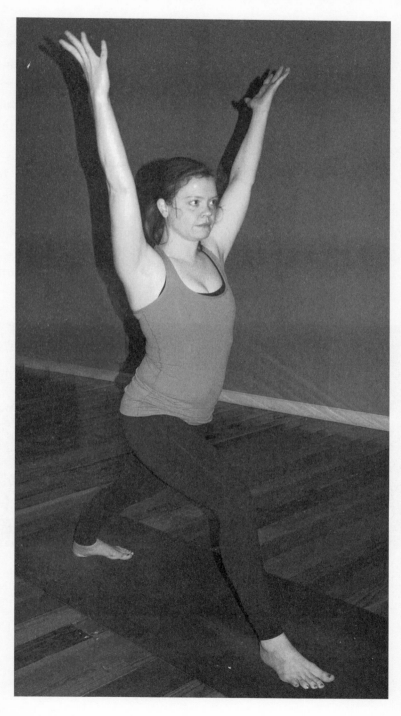

Take a deep inhale, and then exhale to Push-up position.

Lower to floor as you exhale and inhale to Cobra pose. Then exhale back to Downward Facing Dog. Repeat the above steps as follows for the other side. Step your left foot to the front of the mat, and turn your right foot flat for the Warrior 1 pose. Push into your feet as you reach up through your arms, trying to square hips to the front of the room. Take a deep inhale, and then exhale to Push-up position.

Repeat entire Sun Salutation B sequence twice.

Balancing Poses

Modified Side Plank: This pose strengthens your arms and torso, and trains the muscles in your body to work in unison.

Start from the Downward Facing Dog pose. Then pull forward, like you're ready to do a push-up.

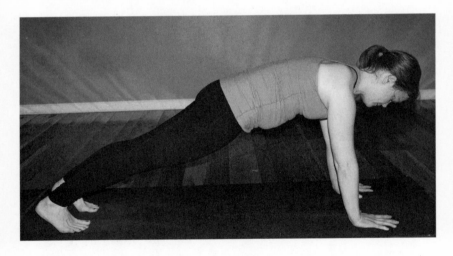

Pull your right knee directly under your right hip.

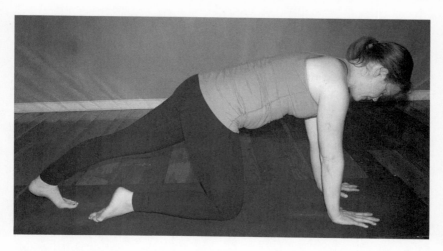

Make sure your right wrist is directly under your right shoulder. Roll onto your right hand and knee as you reach your left arm to the sky. The right hand, knee, and back foot should all be in one line.

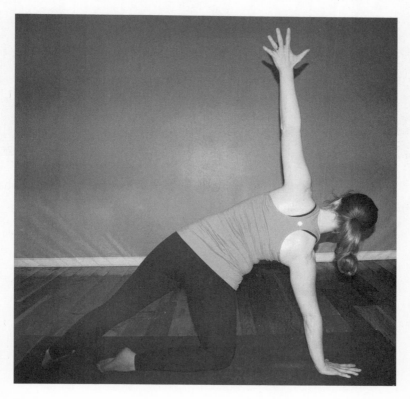

Release to high push-up position, lower yourself to the floor, inhale to Cobra, and exhale to Downward Facing Dog. Then repeat on the left side.

Modified Crescent Lunge: This pose integrates all of your muscles, creating stability in the lower body and lengthening the upper body.

Start from the Downward Facing Dog pose. Step your right foot to your right hand, and drop your left knee to the mat.

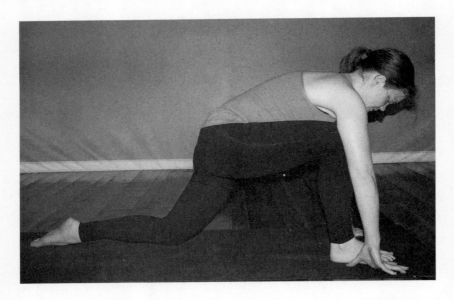

Inhale and reach your arms to the sky as you tuck your tailbone under.

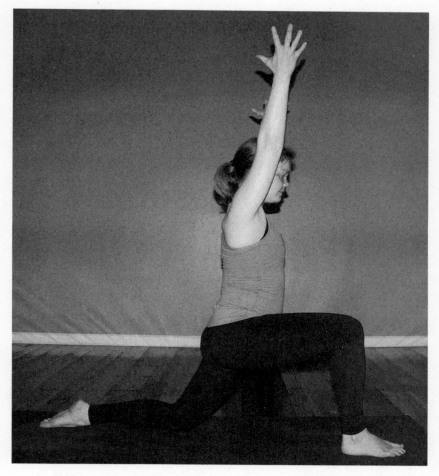

Hold for five breaths. Then return to Push-up position, lower yourself to the floor, inhale to Cobra pose, and exhale to Downward Facing Dog. Repeat these same poses on the left side.

Eagle: The Eagle pose teaches balance and reminds us to center our minds.

Starting from the Downward Facing Dog, step to the front of the mat. Slowly come up to standing and inhale as you reach your arms to the sky. As you exhale, wrap your right arm under your left, bend both knees, and wrap your right leg around your left. Stack your shoulders over your hips, focus your eyes to one point, and hold for five breaths.

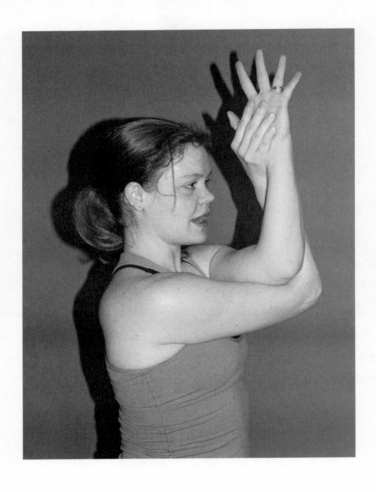

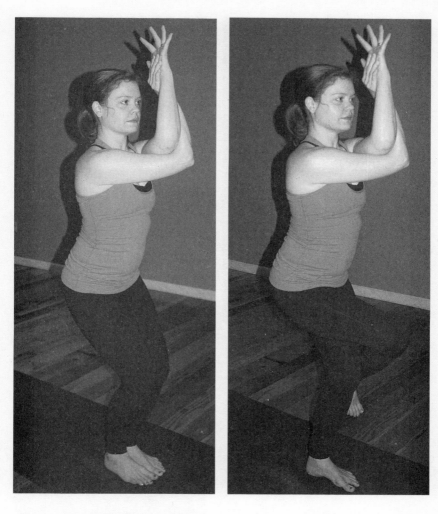

You may modify this by crossing your arms over your shoulders and setting one toe on the floor.

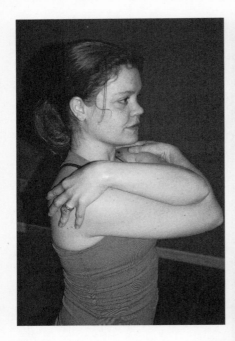

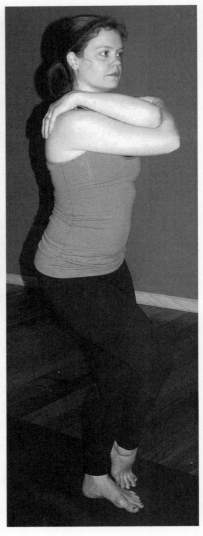

Inhale, reach your arms up to the sky, and then switch to the left side.

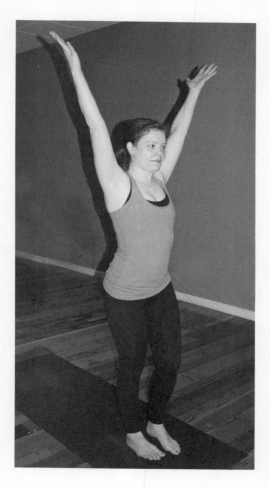

Tree: This still, balancing pose can serve as a standing meditation to bring calm to the body and mind.

Start from standing. Bend your right knee and place the sole of your right foot against the inside of your left leg, being mindful to not press into the knee. Bring your hands to a prayer position at your heart center, gaze at your fingertips for five breaths. Modify this position by placing your right foot at your ankle with your toe touching the floor.

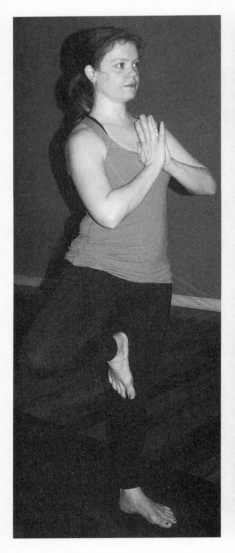
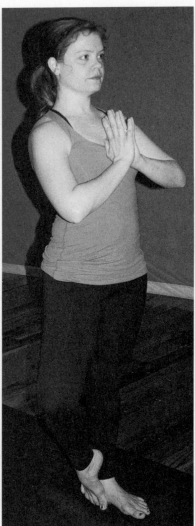

Take five additional breaths, release, and switch to the left side. After the left side, fold forward and step back to Plank position. Lower yourself to the floor, open to Cobra, and press back to Downward Facing Dog.

Floor Poses

Locust: This gentle backbend also stretches out the front of the body.

Start with the Downward Facing Dog, pull forward to Plank position, and yourself lower to the floor. Look down toward your mat and interlace your hands at your tailbone.

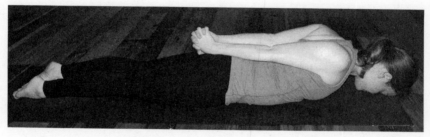

Press your knuckles toward the back of the mat and lift your chest off the mat. Drop your gaze down to release your neck.

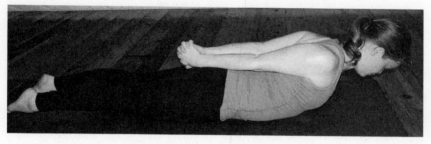

Lift your legs off the mat, pointing back through your toes.

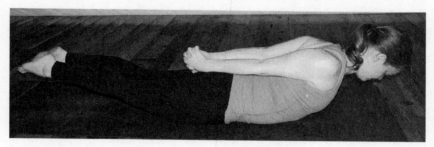

Hold for five breaths and release. Repeat twice, and then move to Downward Facing Dog.

Bridge: This backbend opens the chest and stretches the abdominal wall.

Start from Downward Facing Dog. Step forward, take a seat, and lie back on your mat. Put your feet flat on the mat, with your arms along your sides.

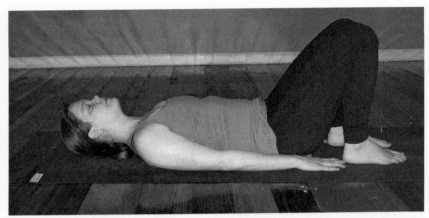

Press down into your feet and hands, and lift your hips off the mat. Make sure your feet are hip-width apart.

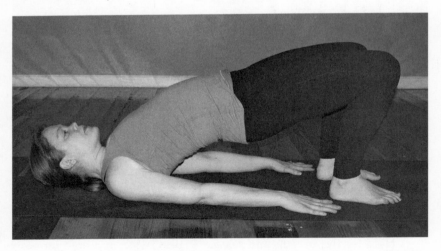

To intensify the posture, interlace your hands under your bridge.

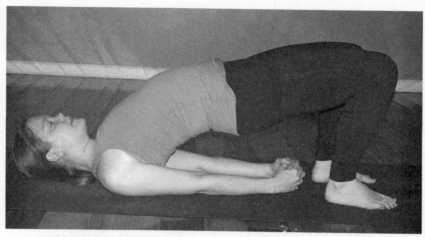

Hold for five breaths and release. Repeat twice.

Reclining Half Pigeon: This deep hip stretch begins to prepare the body for final relaxation.

While still lying on your back with your knees bent, cross your right ankle over your left knee, allowing the right foot to extend to the outside of the left leg.

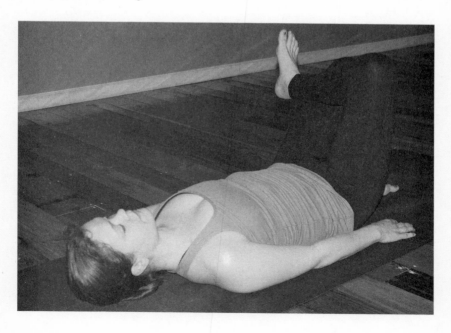

Flex your right toes and grab the back of your left thigh. Gently pull your left knee toward your chest and hold for 5–10 breaths. Release and switch.

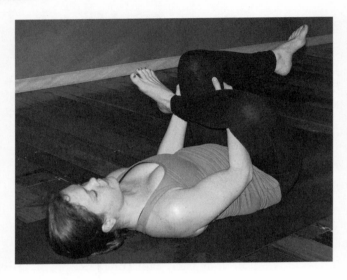

Happy Baby: This position gives a final stretch to the hips, hamstrings, and inner thighs.

Lie on your back and hug your knees into your chest.

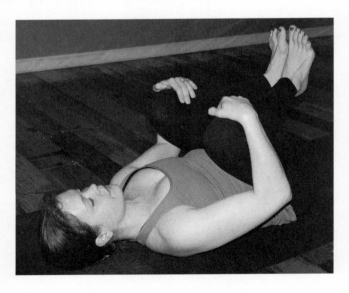

Grab the bottoms of your feet with your hands and draw your knees out and down toward your armpits. The tailbone should be pressing toward the floor, and your head should be relaxed on the mat. Hold for 5–10 breaths and release.

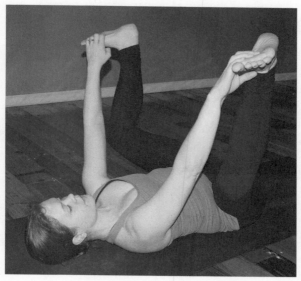

As a modification, push your thighs down instead of holding your feet if your legs feel tight.

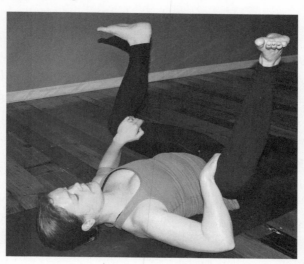

Savasana: Don't skip this final resting pose.

While lying on your back, extend your arms along your sides and your legs long on the mat. Let your entire body just relax into the mat. Feel the relaxation in your face and jaw. Your hands and feet should just relax naturally toward the mat. Allow your body to relax completely and your mind to be quiet for 5 minutes.

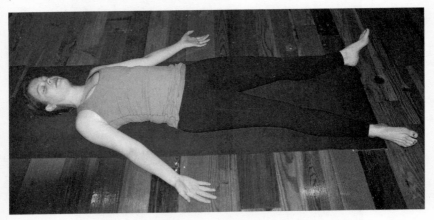

Do you wonder if the meditation aspect of yoga is *really* a valid medical treatment? Researchers from Harvard University published an important study in the journal *Psychiatry Research: Neuroimaging* that helped prove that meditation and mindful yoga resulted in real, measurable changes in the brain. They trained 16 adults in mindful meditation over eight weekly sessions and performed brain scans before and after treatment to look for changes in *gray matter*—the part of the brain that contains nerve cells. Brain scans were also done at the beginning of the study and 8 weeks later in a control group that received no treatment. They found that gray matter increased in several brain regions after completing mindful meditation, including:

▶ The *hippocampus*, a part of the brain that helps control memory and emotion
▶ The *posterior cingulate cortex*, also important for memory and emotion, as well as for pain

- The *temporoparietal junction*, important for interpreting body-related information and sensations and in developing an accurate body image
- The *cerebellum*, important for coordination

There was no change in the hippocampus or temporoparietal gray matter in the control group, with a slight decrease in the posterior cingulate cortex in the no-treatment controls.

This study proved that mindful meditation does more than make you feel emotionally calm. It also helps enhance brain areas important for memory, emotion, and pain.

Meditation needs to be practiced on a regular basis. The more you do it, the greater benefit you will receive.

Psychologist and Pain Specialist
Dr. Dawn Buse Explains How to Meditate

Meditation refers to a group of practices of self-regulation, in which you train your mind to focus attention and awareness to foster general well-being, as well as promote a sense of calm, clarity, and concentration. Meditation has been practiced since antiquity. In modern times, mindful meditation can be used by people with chronic pain and other illnesses to help manage stress and enhance health. Mindfulness focuses on experiencing each moment fully and nonjudgmentally; this is often referred to as "being in the present moment." Focused awareness is a primary component of all forms of meditation.

To get started, find a quiet environment that is free of distractions and make yourself as comfortable as possible. Sit in a chair or lie on the floor. Loosen or remove any tight-fitting clothes, such as belts or shoes. Reduce outside noise and turn off your cell phone. You may want to set an alarm so you will not be tempted to keep looking at your watch or a clock during meditation. Start by meditating for 15–20 minutes at each session.

- Relax any muscles in your body that feel tight. Some people like to start with a progressive muscle relaxation exercise. (See Chapter 7.)

(continued on next page)

▶ Close your eyes and focus on your breath. Breathe in through your nose, and out through your mouth. As you exhale, really push the air out, using your diaphragm and making a soft "whooshing" sound.

▶ Once you have achieved a deep and steady state of breathing (choosing a pace that is slow but comfortable), you may want to add a mantra, which is a calming word (such as "ohm" or "peace") that you say with each breath, either silently or out loud. Choose a word that has a positive meaning for you. The more you practice using a mantra, the more it will produce the conditioned response of relaxation and bring greater peace and calm. You might prefer to count silently to yourself as you inhale and exhale. Breathe easily and naturally.

▶ Do not worry about whether you are meditating "right," or whether you will be successful in achieving a deep state of relaxation. Maintain a nonjudgmental and passive attitude, and permit the meditation and relaxation to occur at its own pace. When distracting thoughts occur (as they will), simply return your focus to your breath, counting, or repetition of your mantra. Imagine that each distracting thought is like a cloud that simply floats across the sky. The thought may come into your mind, but just like the breeze pushes a cloud across the sky, it also floats out on its own.

▶ Continue meditating for the amount of time you have set. When you have finished, sit quietly for several minutes—at first with your eyes closed, and then with your eyes open. Allow yourself to enjoy the deep feelings of relaxation in your body. Practice meditation on a daily basis or any other schedule you prefer.

Tai Chi

Tai chi is a mind–body therapy that combines meditation with slow, graceful movements, deep breathing, and relaxation. It is well established as an effective therapy for reducing pain related to arthritis. Tai chi also improves cardiovascular health, sleep, energy, balance, and mood, and promotes a feeling of well-being. It should be taught by a qualified Tai chi instructor, so that you learn how to do the exercises correctly.

A well-designed study tested the benefits for people with fibromyalgia of Tai chi taught by a master for 60-minute sessions, twice a week for 12 weeks. In addition to these classes, participants were instructed to practice stretching at home for 20 minutes each day. After completing this treatment, the participants' pain levels were reduced by 43 percent, disability decreased by 44 percent, sleep improved by 26 percent, and mood improved by 36 percent. These benefits were still present when the participants were examined 3 months later.

MASSAGE

Limited research has been done evaluating the benefits of different types of massage for people with fibromyalgia. Each of the massage techniques found to be helpful and that are described below are administered by trained physical therapists.

- ▶ Manual lymph drainage
  - For this massage, the therapist applies gentle, rhythmic pressure to different parts of the body to massage the lymph vessels, which helps push fluid though the lymph system.
- ▶ Connective tissue massage
  - Connective tissues are the body's support network that hold all the organs and the body together.
  - For this massage, the therapist stretches connective tissue close to the skin to reduce tension in the autonomic nervous system, which improves circulation, muscle relaxation, and mobility.
- ▶ Myofascial release
  - *Myo* is the medical term for muscles and *fascia* are tissues covering muscles.
  - For this massage, the therapist massages and stretches muscles and fascia to reduce muscle tension. These techniques are

designed to relax muscles, increase lymph drainage, and improve circulation.

Potential benefits from other types of massage have not been tested in fibromyalgia patients.

Research suggests that massage may help fibromyalgia by reducing the release of chemicals, called *neurotransmitters*, that transmit pain signals from the body to the brain. One study treated people with fibromyalgia for 30 minutes twice a week for 5 weeks with either massage therapy or relaxation training. Mood improved in both groups, while pain was also reduced in the group that received massage. Levels of *substance P*, an important pain neurotransmitter, were also reduced in this group, thus supporting a biological basis for massage therapy.

ACUPUNCTURE

Acupuncture is helpful for several chronic pain conditions, including musculoskeletal pain in the neck, shoulder, elbow, and low back resulting from soft tissue injuries and arthritis. It may also help relieve tension-type headaches. However, acupuncture does not seem to help reduce the pain associated with fibromyalgia. A recent analysis of data from six well-designed research studies that tested acupuncture in a total of 323 people with fibromyalgia showed that it did not significantly improve pain severity.

Acupuncture has been shown to improve insomnia, although not specifically in people with fibromyalgia. It has also been used to treat irritable bowel syndrome, although benefits have been inconsistent.

SUMMARY

▶ Non-drug therapies are effective for relieving the symptoms of fibromyalgia.

▶ Aerobic and strengthening exercises are some of the most effective non-medication therapies, especially if they are performed consistently and preceded by stretching.

▶ Yoga can be quite helpful for people with fibromyalgia because it combines strength training and relaxation. Yoga combined with meditation can be even more helpful.

▶ Exercising in a warm pool may increase its benefits.

▶ Modest benefits may be achieved with massage.

▶ Acupuncture is generally ineffective for fibromyalgia pain, although it may help relieve other symptoms.

7

Behavioral Strategies and
Lifestyle Changes
for Fibromyalgia

Non-drug treatments, such as behavioral therapies, relaxation, and stress management, are real, biologically based therapies that help change the way the brain experiences, interprets, and sends pain messages. They help you learn to use the power of your brain to change the way it interprets and responds to different nerve signals and blocks pain messages. Improvement in fibromyalgia symptoms from psychological treatments does *not* mean that fibromyalgia is a mental or emotional disorder. If you have a serious psychological problem—for example, severe depression or anxiety—you will probably not get much benefit from psychological pain management techniques until your mood is under better control.

BEHAVIORAL THERAPIES

When people think about working with a psychologist, they often think of *psychotherapy*, which is sometimes called *talk therapy*. Psychotherapy focuses on understanding conflicts and problems that contribute to emotional distress—it enables you to understand *why* you feel

Cognitive-Behavioral Therapy Changes
How You Think About Your Pain

▶ *Change your thoughts from negative to positive.* Negative thoughts about fibromyalgia include catastrophic thinking that the pain will never improve, that nothing you can do will help, and that achieving pain relief is hopeless. Typical negative thoughts might be:
- "I'll never get better."
- "It's hopeless."
- "I'm doomed to spend my days on the couch."
- "Nothing I do for pain makes a difference."

▶ *Cognitive-behavioral therapy teaches you to give yourself positive messages.*
- "I'm taking control of my fibromyalgia, one day at a time."
- "If I take a break and practice some pain techniques, my pain level will become more manageable."
- "I'll schedule my activities more carefully so I don't do too much and get wiped out."
- "Sticking with my exercise program will help reduce my disability."

▶ *Set realistic goals.* Don't expect your treatment to cure your fibromyalgia. Realistic goals might include:
- Decrease pain severity from severe to moderate
- Decrease the time you spend in bed or lying on the sofa
- Increase your ability to do household chores and attend family activities and social functions
- Reduce problems with mood or anxiety
- Improve sleep
- Improve bowel function
- Reduce your reliance on medications

Try setting specific goals for yourself. Instead of "wanting to be more active," set targets such as "being able to shop for 20 minutes," "being able to walk 20 minutes each day," and "being able to cook dinner for the family."

▶ *Schedule your tasks for success.* You'll be more successful if you break tasks into smaller segments. For example, if you want to do the laundry, load and run the machine in the morning, then do your stretching exercises, followed by a 10-minute walk. Switch clothes to the dryer in the afternoon and practice some deep breathing. Finally, fold the clothes while sitting down watching television in the evening. If you break tasks down and take breaks between segments, it will be easier to accomplish your goals.

depressed or anxious. Openly sharing your difficulties with a therapist can be a good way to develop insights into personal issues and take an important first step toward recovery. However, this is not what we mean when we discuss using behavioral therapy to help manage fibromyalgia.

Instead of focusing on understanding the root of a problem, *behavioral therapy* focuses on changing your behavior to relieve your symptoms. This therapy focuses on learning techniques that can reduce your symptoms, rather than the reasons for your distress. Behavioral therapy skills are among the most effective techniques for reducing a wide range of chronic pain conditions, including fibromyalgia, migraine, and others.

The most effective psychological treatments for fibromyalgia are *cognitive-behavioral therapy* and *conditioning behavioral therapy* (also called *operant-behavioral therapy*). Cognitive-behavioral therapy changes the way you *think* about fibromyalgia. It helps you reduce negative thoughts that can make your symptoms worse. Conditioning behavioral therapy can change how you *react* to pain by helping you reduce behaviors that may increase your pain.

Cognitive-behavioral and conditioning behavioral therapies are among the most effective fibromyalgia treatments. For example, in one well-designed study, 125 people with fibromyalgia were randomly assigned to treatment with cognitive-behavioral therapy, conditioning behavioral therapy, or to a control group that received no skills training. Skills were taught in groups of five patients, seen for 2-hour sessions once a week for 15 weeks. The control group received general education without any specific training. One year after treatment, people getting either treatment improved more than the control group. In addition:

> *Conditioning behavioral therapy can change how you react to pain by helping you reduce behaviors that may increase your pain.*

- ▶ Pain levels dropped by at least half in 45 percent of those treated with cognitive-behavioral therapy and 54 percent of those who

Conditioning Behavioral Therapy Changes How You *Act* When You Experience Pain

When we have pain, we often talk about it and moan, grimace, or move our bodies differently. When other people see and hear us, they respond to our pain behaviors. Sometimes, these responses can encourage you to do things that won't really help your symptoms. For example, some people may talk about how bad their own pain is, or encourage you to take extra pain pills, go to bed, or call the doctor. People may also add to your negative thinking by saying such things as, "Your fibromyalgia always interferes with our fun" or "Every time we try to do something, fibromyalgia gets in the way."

Conditioning behavioral therapy trains you to avoid displaying as many pain behaviors; for example:

▶ Pay attention to how much you talk about your pain with others and try to shift conversations to more positive topics.

▶ Watch how you move and walk when your symptoms are bothering you, and try to move more normally.

▶ Catch yourself when you hear yourself moaning or groaning as you move.

Conditioning behavioral therapy also trains others to encourage you in doing the things your doctor has recommended. Positive behaviors could include:

▶ Tell your family and friends, "Let's not talk about my pain. What's new with you?"

▶ Let them know that you need encouragement to be active, and request that they suggest activities that keep you moving.

▶ Remind family and friends that you want to keep up with your chores, so that they'd don't jump in and finish them for you.

▶ Ask them to suggest fun activities to help distract you from your symptoms.

received conditioning behavioral therapy, but in only 5 percent of the control group.

▶ Disability decreased by at least half for 38 percent treated with cognitive-behavioral therapy and for 58 percent with conditioning behavioral therapy, but for only 8 percent of the control group.

▶ The number of physician visits dropped by 17 percent after cognitive-behavioral therapy and by 56 percent with conditioning behavioral therapy. In contrast, visits increased by 39 percent in the control group.

RELAXATION TECHNIQUES

Relaxation techniques can help reduce pain levels and other symptoms of fibromyalgia. They are most helpful when combined with other pain management techniques, such as cognitive-behavioral therapy. Several effective techniques for relaxation are described here to help you get started.

When you are learning a new relaxation technique, sit in a comfortable chair in a quiet room. Don't cross your arms or legs, and make sure your feet are resting flat on the floor. Close your eyes and begin the exercises. While you are first learning these techniques, practice them once or twice a day for 15–20 minutes, hopefully at a time when your symptoms are mild. Once you have regularly practiced and mastered the techniques, you will be able to achieve deeper states of relaxation during your 15–20-minute sessions. You also will be able to practice mini-relaxation sessions whenever you feel an increase in stress, anxiety, or pain.

As with any skill, you will need to practice for a while before you feel comfortable with the exercises, and they are consistently helpful when your stress or pain levels are high. Working with a behavioral psychologist can help you master these skills. Use the following techniques suggested by Dawn Buse, a psychologist and assistant professor at Albert Einstein College of Medicine, to help you start learning to relax.

How Does Relaxation Reduce Pain?

The brain and nervous system keep your body in balance via the *sympathetic* and *parasympathetic* nerves. The sympathetic nerves provide activation, and the parasympathetic nerves cause relaxation. When we experience stress or danger, the sympathetic system goes into overdrive to prepare the body for action. This is called the "fight-or-flight" response. Activation by the sympathetic nerves gets us ready for action—to do battle or to run away from it. When this happens, your heart beats faster, your blood pressure rises, and your breathing becomes faster and more shallow. You begin to sweat, which helps cool down your body. Blood flow is moved away from your skin and into your deeper muscles. As a result, your muscles get more of the available blood and oxygen, and your hands and feet will feel cold and clammy. Blood is also diverted away from your digestive tract, which can cause stomach pain, constipation, or diarrhea. These changes all help prepare the body for action—to fight or run away from danger.

These involuntary fight-or-flight responses are helpful when experiencing a physical threat—for example, they helped our distant ancestors survive. However, many stresses in modern life aren't dealt with by fighting or fleeing. If your boss is critiquing your latest work project, or your teenager is negotiating for the family car, you'll likely experience a stress response. But you are unlikely to start a physical battle or dash out of the room. The physical responses that would be helpful if we met a bear in the woods aren't really helpful at home or in the boardroom!

When we experience frequent stressful situations, the constant activation of the sympathetic nervous system produces a significant negative effect on the body. Repeated stress can affect the immune system, make us more prone to becoming overweight, cause fatigue, affect our ability to concentrate, and put stress on the heart and gastrointestinal systems. These responses can, in turn, aggravate pain, such as the pain caused by fibromyalgia.

Fortunately, we can avoid long-term damage from chronic fight-or-flight responses by learning to activate the parasympathetic system. The relaxation it produces balances out the activation of the fight-or-flight response and allows your body to release chemicals and brain signals that reverse the effects caused by the sympathetic nervous system. Relaxation also helps turn off the activation of pain signals. When you achieve deep relaxation, your:

▶ Breathing becomes slow, deep, and regular
▶ Heart rate slows down
▶ Blood returns to your skin so that your hands and feet feel warmer
▶ Muscle tension is reduced

Relaxation can be achieved through a wide range of techniques, including:

▶ Deep, diaphragmatic breathing
▶ Visual imagery
▶ Progressive muscle relaxation
▶ Cue-controlled relaxation
▶ Yoga
▶ Prayer or meditation
▶ Listening to calming or pleasant music
▶ Petting a cat or dog

Deep, Diaphragmatic Breathing

This type of breathing involves becoming consciously aware you are taking slow, deep breaths. The diaphragm is a sheet of muscle at the base of the lungs that helps expand the lungs and pull in oxygen when you breathe in—and push air out when you breathe out. The technique involves shifting from the rapid, shallow, and anxious breathing that occurs when you're feeling stressed, to deep breathing that uses the diaphragm more effectively. To breathe effectively in this way:

▶ Place one hand on your chest and one on your abdomen.
▶ Pay attention to which hand is moving as you take each breath. When you take stressful shallow breaths, your *chest* will move more as you breathe. With deep, relaxing breaths, your *abdomen* will move more.

▶ Therefore, you should breathe slowly and evenly, so that the hand over your abdomen moves more than the one over your chest.

▶ Breathe in slowly and deeply through your nose, attempting to move the hand on your abdomen as if you were inflating a balloon. Your chest should only move slightly, and only when your abdomen also moves.

▶ After you inhale, count to four. Then, gently exhale through your mouth, making a soft whooshing sound as you breathe out.

▶ Allow your mouth, tongue, and jaw to feel loose and relaxed.

▶ Continue to take long, slow, deep breaths that raise and lower your abdomen. If your attention begins to wander, try counting while you breathe or repeat the word "calm" with each breath.

Visual Imagery

Visual imagery builds on deep-breathing practice by adding a mental picture that can improve your sense of calmness, peace, safety, and tranquility. To practice visual imagery:

▶ First, do deep or diaphragmatic breathing for a few minutes, focusing on expanding your lungs like a balloon, then gently exhaling through your mouth with a soft, whooshing sound.

▶ Think of a beautiful, peaceful scene, such as a warm tropical beach, a fragrant meadow, or a mountain stream, or perhaps sitting by a roaring fire in a mountain cabin or soaring in a hot air balloon. Choose a place you've been before, or imagine one you've never experienced. Use the same location every time you do this relaxation practice.

▶ Once you've chosen a location, use each of your senses to imagine you are really there. For example, if you choose a tropical sunny beach, imagine how it looks. What are you wearing? Are you wearing shoes or barefoot? A sun hat? Are you walking along the water, lying in a hammock under a palm tree, or relaxing on a chaise lounge? Imagine the color and texture of the sand beneath your feet. Is it warm or hot? Is the water cool? Look at the beautiful blues and greens of the water, the size of the waves, and the blue of the sky. Are there clouds, birds, trees, boats, or anything else in your ideal scene? Once you have "looked around," notice the tangy scent of the ocean, the droplets of spray when the waves crash on the shore, the scent of your suntan lotion, and the feel of the warm sun on your arms and face. Use all of your senses to imagine yourself in your chosen setting, and then allow yourself to feel peaceful, tranquil, and relaxed.

▶ Tell yourself that you are calm and relaxed, peaceful and safe.

▶ Notice the feelings of heaviness in your arms and legs, and the warmth in your hands. As you relax deeper into the image, your arms and legs should feel heavy and relaxed, and your arms and feet should become warmer.

Progressive Muscle Relaxation

This technique involves contracting and then relaxing muscles throughout your body:

▶ Close your eyes.

▶ Practice tensing then relaxing individual muscles. Tense and release the muscles in your feet, then work upward into your legs, abdomen, hands, arms, shoulders, neck, jaw, eyes, and forehead.

▶ Hold the tension in each muscle for 10–15 seconds and then release it.

▶ Focus on how the muscles feel when they are no longer tensed.

After you've practiced this exercise a few times, you'll begin to recognize when your muscles first get tense. As you feel them becoming tense, take a few minutes and practice progressive muscle relaxation.

Cue-Controlled Relaxation

This technique involves deep breathing while repeating the word "relax." Eventually, this word will become your "cue" to relax.

▶ Take a slow, deep, abdominal breath.

▶ To make sure you're doing abdominal breathing, place your hand over your abdomen when you breathe. Feel it move in and out with each deep breath.

▶ After breathing in, hold your breath for 5–10 seconds. Then slowly exhale and repeat the word "relax" as you blow out air. Repeat.

▶ When you've practiced this exercise a number of times, try closing your eyes and taking deep abdominal breaths *before* dealing with a stressful situation. First, try this exercise while you are standing in the shower, then while waiting in line at a store, before talking to your teenager or spouse, or before meeting with your boss or your child's teacher. You can also use cue-controlled relaxation when you start to feel stressed or your fibromyalgia symptoms worsen.

STRESS MANAGEMENT

Stress is an important trigger for many medical symptoms, including chronic pain. Studies in both animals and humans prove that reactions to stress can actually make us more sensitive to painful stimulation. When you're under stress, you may notice more fibromyalgia symptoms and less reserve to tolerate them. Stress management can reduce your symptoms, although the effects will not be as substantial as those seen with aerobic exercise. In general, stress management techniques should be combined with other fibromyalgia treatments.

Men and women respond differently to stress. Changes in brain chemicals—including chemicals important for managing pain, such as serotonin, dopamine, and acetylcholine—are different whether you're a man or woman. The effects of stress on memory, learning, and per-

Stress Busting Techniques

▶ *Learn good time management.* Schedule a reasonable number of activities, chores, or goals for each day. Overloading your schedule will inevitably result in a stress response:

- Write down which activities must be completed each day, and delegate chores among the members of your household.

- Accept that life won't be perfect. It's more important to have a relaxed home than a spotless house.

- Don't be afraid to say "no." You can't volunteer for every worthwhile cause, and your kids don't need to participate in every possible after-school activity. Prioritize what's important for you and your family. Research shows that it is healthiest to limit volunteer activities to no more than 2 hours per week.

- Schedule "down time" every day for reading, reflection, or a fun family activity.

▶ *Identify your stress buttons.* Learn what events typically make you feel stressed. For example, you might be stressed after a meeting with your boss, while helping with a school project, or talking with your mother-in-law:

- Anticipate your stress triggers, and practice relaxation techniques and telling yourself positive, affirming messages before encountering stress.

- Stretch your muscles when they first become tense.

- Give yourself positive, encouraging messages before beginning any stressful activity.

▶ *Practice daily stress-busting.*

- Recognize and accept stressful events you can't control (for example, the weather or other people's attitudes and behavior).

- Ask for help from others—you don't have to do everything yourself!

- Do aerobic exercise every day.

- Consider learning and practicing yoga, Tai chi, and/or mindfulness meditation.

- Eat regularly—don't skip meals.

- Get plenty of sleep.

- Sing and find humor in your day.

formance are also different in men and women. In one interesting study, stress effects were measured in men and women after viewing a disturbing video. Although the effects were similar for both the first time the video was watched, repeated viewing resulted in more negative effects in the women. This suggests that women are more vulnerable to negative health effects from chronic exposure to stress, compared with men. For this reason, regular use of stress management techniques to reduce the impact of stress may be particularly important for women.

HEALTHY LIFESTYLE HABITS

When you have fibromyalgia, you don't need additional health problems caused by unhealthy lifestyle habits. Taking care of yourself by controlling your weight, getting sufficient sleep, eating right, and avoiding unhealthy habits such as smoking is important for your overall health and for managing fibromyalgia. In addition, unhealthy lifestyle habits can aggravate your symptoms. It's important for everyone to follow healthy lifestyle habits, but this is even more important when you have fibromyalgia.

Weight Management

Obesity is a global epidemic that affects approximately one-quarter of adults in the United States and Europe, and one-fifth of adults in China. Obesity is generally defined as weighing 20 percent or more over your ideal body weight. Being overweight is even more common among people with fibromyalgia. Seven in every ten people with fibromyalgia are overweight, and half can be classified as obese.

Most doctors define overweight and obesity using the *body mass index* (BMI), which takes into consideration your weight in relation to your height. A normal BMI is less than 25. BMIs between 25 and 29.9 show that you're overweight. If your BMI is 30 or higher, you are obese, meaning you have a serious and unhealthy amount of excess weight. For example, if you are 5 feet 9 inches tall, your healthy weight would be approximately 125–168 pounds. Between 169–202 pounds, you'd be considered overweight, and if you weigh over 202 pounds you would be considered obese. BMI calculators on the Internet can calculate this for you—a good one, sponsored by the National Heart, Lung, and Blood Institute, can be found at http://www.nhlbisupport.com/bmi/.

Obesity is more than a cosmetic problem. It increases the risk of developing a variety of health conditions, including heart disease, diabetes, lung diseases, arthritis, fatty liver, gallbladder disease, reproductive problems, skin conditions, and cancer. A survey of 100 randomly selected people with fibromyalgia also found that those who were obese were:

- ▶ More sensitive to pain
- ▶ More likely to be out of shape
- ▶ More likely to have a poorer quality of life

Losing weight should substantially improve your fibromyalgia pain. In a 20-week study conducted at the University of Albany, overweight and obese people with fibromyalgia were treated using a weight loss program

Strategies for Successful Weight Loss

- ▶ Exercise 30 minutes daily.
- ▶ Add physical activity to daily life.
- ▶ Avoid over-the-counter diet pills.
- ▶ Plan meals.
- ▶ Count calories and measure the fat content of foods.
- ▶ Measure portion sizes.
- ▶ Weigh yourself daily.

(Based on Kruger 2006; see References)

that focused on dietary restrictions and increased physical activity, including 30 minutes of daily aerobic exercise. Participants lost an average of a little more than 9 pounds, and their pain, disability, and mood disturbances improved significantly. Another study that treated morbidly obese people with fibromyalgia using weight loss surgery reported substantial reductions in weight, severity of pain, and medication use.

Sleep Management

Poor sleep increases your risk of becoming obese and developing diabetes, because sleep helps curb your appetite and control glucose metabolism. People with poor sleep also have higher levels of inflammatory chemicals that can increase their risk for high blood pressure and heart disease. Interestingly, sleep is also linked to pain sensitivity. People with poor sleep have a lower pain threshold, so your pain will be more severe when you're sleeping poorly.

How much sleep do you need? Adults typically need 7–9 hours of sleep each night for good health. Unfortunately, most people with fibromyalgia have problems with sleep. Getting better sleep will help make your other pain treatments more effective.

Make sure you tell your doctor about any sleep problems you may be having. A good way to rate your sleep is to use the *Sleep Quality Scale*:

Rate your sleep quality over the last 24 hours from zero to ten	
0 = best possible sleep	10 = worst possible sleep

Your doctor can suggest a variety of changes that might improve the quality of your sleep. Occasionally, you may need medications to help regulate your sleep. Talk to your doctor about medications that have also been shown to reduce other fibromyalgia symptoms:

▶ Antidepressants: duloxetine (Cymbalta®), milnacipran (Savella®), and amitriptyline (Elavil®)

Practice These Good Sleep Habits

▶ Daily habits to help with sleep:

- Avoid excessive daytime napping; don't nap more than once each afternoon or for longer than 45 minutes.
- Do aerobic exercise daily.

▶ Prepare for better sleep:

- Reduce evening stimulants, such as caffeine and nicotine.
- Don't drink alcohol before going to bed.
- Practice relaxation techniques at bedtime.
- Avoid stimulating activities for several hours before bed.
- Dim ambient lighting 1–2 hours before bed to prepare for sleep.
- Eat a light evening snack before bed, such as a bowl of cereal or glass of milk.
- Make sure your bedroom is pleasantly cool.

▶ Bedtime habits:

- Establish and maintain regular sleep and rise times.
- Use your bed only for sleep and sex.
- Go to bed only when you are sleepy.
- Don't watch television or read in bed.
- If too much ambient light enters the bedroom, an eye mask may be helpful.
- If noise in the bedroom prevents sleep, try using earplugs.
- If you are unable to fall asleep after 15 minutes, get up and go to another room.
- Only return to bed when you are sleepy.

▶ Antiepileptic drugs: pregabalin (Lyrica®) and gabapentin (Neurontin®)

▶ Sleep disorder drug: sodium oxybate (Xyrem®)

Diet

Several dietary regimens previously recommended for fibromyalgia have shown no benefits, including supplementation with soy shakes and weekly intravenous nutrient therapy that included minerals and vitamins (the so-called the *Myers' cocktail*).

Nutritional therapy may be helpful for reducing digestive symptoms that result from irritable bowel disease, but it's important to distinguish irritable bowel syndrome (IBS) from *celiac disease*, an inherited autoimmune disease that causes a variety of unpleasant digestive symptoms, including pain, bloating, diarrhea, and constipation. It may also cause pain, fatigue, and mood disturbance, thus further mimicking fibromyalgia. Celiac disease is treated with a gluten-free diet.

Effective Dietary Treatments for Irritable Bowel Syndrome (IBS)

▶ Fiber therapy:
  - Increasing soluble fiber improves constipation and other irritable bowel symptoms but not abdominal pain.

▶ Peppermint oil:
  - Three to six enteric-coated capsules containing 0.2–0.4 mL peppermint oil daily can reduce irritable bowel symptoms, including abdominal pain. Capsules need to be swallowed and not chewed to avoid reflux.

▶ Herbs:
  - Tong xie yao fang, Padma Lax, and STW 5 have been found to reduce the symptoms of IBS.

▶ Probiotics:
  - Probiotic supplements or eating more foods rich in probiotics (such as yogurt, kefir [fermented milk], miso and tempeh made from soybeans, and sauerkraut) relieves irritable bowel symptoms and abdominal pain.

Stop Smoking

Approximately one in four people with fibromyalgia smokes. Using nicotine changes a number of important brain chemicals that affect pain, including endorphins, serotonin, norepinephrine, and dopamine. These nicotine-induced changes in brain chemicals make you more sensitive to pain. In an interesting study of 984 people with fibromyalgia at the Mayo Clinic, pain and disability were both significantly worse among those who were smokers. In addition, problems with work, sleep, stiffness, anxiety, and depression were all significantly more impaired among participants who used tobacco. A similar Korean study of 336 people with fibromyalgia found a link between smoking status and pain, functional disability, and mood. Although smoking doesn't *cause* fibromyalgia, it generally worsens the severity of chronic pain conditions, including fibromyalgia.

Smoking can also decrease the effectiveness of pain medications:

▶ Smokers use more painkillers than do non-smokers.
▶ When taking the same amount of painkillers, blood concentrations are lower in smokers.
▶ Smokers get less pain relief from taking pain medication.

Smoking may reduce the effectiveness of antidepressants. Smokers taking antidepressants to treat mood problems experience less of an improvement, as compared with non-smokers using the same drugs.

SUMMARY

▶ Cognitive- and conditioning-behavioral therapies are effective techniques for reducing fibromyalgia symptoms.
▶ Relaxation techniques and stress management are moderately helpful for fibromyalgia.
▶ Lifestyle modifications, including smoking cessation, sleep regulation, and weight management, are important for improved general health, with some fibromyalgia-specific symptom benefits also expected.

8

What Medications Really Help and Which Ones Don't

Fibromyalgia treatment is not an either-or proposition. You don't need to use *either* medications *or* non-drug treatments, and you don't need to use *either* medications prescribed by your doctor *or* natural supplements. Medications are usually best used to complement and supplement effective non-drug treatments. The most effective fibromyalgia treatment regimen often uses *combination therapy*—which combines non-drug and drug therapies.

Tell your doctor about all of the medications you use—including over-the-counter, prescription, and nutritional therapies.

Just like non-drug treatments, you will probably need to try several medications before your find the right drugs, dosage, and combination for you. Tell your doctor about *all* of the medications you use—including over-the-counter, prescription, and nutritional therapies.

MEDICATIONS USED TO MANAGE FIBROMYALGIA

A number of medications can be used to help relieve a range of fibromyalgia symptoms. For example, antidepressants may reduce pain, sleep disturbance, depression, and some digestive symptoms. You may

MEDICATIONS FOR MIGRAINE*

Infrequent Migraines Typically Occurring Less Than 3 Days Per Week		Frequent Migraines Typically Occurring 3 or More Days Per Week Need Prevention Therapies	
Drug Category	**Examples**	**Drug Category**	**Examples**
Analgesics	Aspirin Acetaminophen Ibuprofen Naproxen	Antidepressants	Amitriptyline (Elavil®) Imipramine (Tofranil®)
Analgesics plus caffeine	Excedrin® Ibuprofen plus 1/2 can of cola	Neuromodulating therapies	Topiramate (Topamax®) Valproate (Depakote®) Gabapentin (Neurontin®)
Triptan	Sumatriptan Rizatriptan (Maxalt®) Eletriptan (Relpax®) Zolmitriptan (Zomig®) Almotriptan (Axert®)	Blood pressure medications	Timolol (Blocadren®) Propranolol (Inderal®) Verapamil (Calan®)
Ergotamine	Dihydroergotamine		*Drugs that reduce migraine frequency were initially tested for other health conditions. Effective migraine prevention drugs include therapies initially designed to improve mood, nerve diseases, and high blood pressure.*
Antinausea medication	Metoclopramide (Reglan®) Promethazine (Phenergan®) Prochlorperazine (Compazine®)		

*More information on managing migraines can be found in *The Woman's Migraine Toolkit*.

also need to use specific therapies for some symptoms, such as severe depression or anxiety, migraine, or irritable bowel syndrome (IBS).

The most important thing to remember about medications for fibromyalgia is that even the most effective ones offer modest benefit at best:

MEDICATIONS FOR IRRITABLE BOWEL SYNDROME (IBS)

Medication	Condition Improved	Significant Side Effects
Serotonin (5HT) receptor agents		
5HT$_3$ antagonist alosetron (Lotronex®)	Global IBS symptoms in women with diarrhea	Constipation
Antidepressants		
Tricyclic	Abdominal pain	Constipation
SSRI	Abdominal pain	Better tolerated than tricyclics
Gastrointestinal agents		
Loperamide (Imodium®)	Diarrhea	Constipation
Fiber/bulking agents	Constipation	Bloating
Oral cromolyn sodium	Diarrhea	Constipation
Selective chloride channel-2 activator lubiprostone (Amitiza®)	Constipation	Nausea Diarrhea Headache

▶ Effective medications should be expected to reduce fibromyalgia pain and other symptoms by about 30 percent.

▶ Because symptom reduction with drugs is modest to moderate, medications should generally be used in conjunction with effective non-drug treatments.

▶ The most effective medications for fibromyalgia are antidepressants and some neuromodulating therapies. Both types of drugs work by correcting chemical imbalances in nerve chemicals within the nervous system, to help reduce fibromyalgia symptoms.

▶ Antidepressants and neuromodulating therapies reduce pain and poor sleep. Antidepressants are more beneficial for also reducing fatigue and mood problems.

Antidepressants

A variety of antidepressants may help reduce fibromyalgia symptoms, but the most effective ones are the *serotonin norepinephrine reuptake inhibitor* (SNRI) antidepressants, including duloxetine (Cymbalta®) and milnacipran (Savella®). The tricyclic antidepressant amitriptyline (Elavil®) is also moderately helpful, although it has substantially more side effects than the SNRI antidepressants for most people. Selective serotonin reuptake inhibitors (SSRIs, such as paroxetine [Paxil®] and fluoxetine [Prozac®] are generally less effective for reducing fibromyalgia symptoms than SNRI or tricyclic antidepressants.

Neuromodulating Therapies

Neuromodulating drugs modify the level of activation of different nerves in the brain, by decreasing abnormal activity in the nervous system. Most neuromodulating drugs were initially designed to reduce the abnormal brain signaling that can produce seizures in people who have epilepsy. Physicians later found that many of the same drugs that blocked seizures could also reduce the number of pain signals being sent in the nervous systems of people with some chronic pain conditions. Neuromodulating drugs are commonly used to reduce symptoms for people with nerve pain, such as neuropathy, migraines, and fibromyalgia.

Pregabalin (Lyrica®) and gabapentin (Neurontin®) are two neuromodulating drugs that have been shown to improve pain, disability, and sleep disturbance in people with fibromyalgia. They also reduce digestive system hypersensitivity, and may help reduce irritable bowel symptoms.

Sleep Medications

Although some sleep medications may offer short-term improvement, sleep disturbances are better treated with drugs that have a strong track record for long-term use in fibromyalgia and that may help relieve more symptoms than just poor sleep. The medications most consistently found to improve fibromyalgia pain and sleep disturbance include antidepressants, pregabalin (Lyrica®), and gabapentin (Neurontin®). Tizanidine (Zanaflex®) reduces pain and sleep disturbance in people with spasms and muscular pain, and it may also be helpful in fibromyalgia.

Sodium oxybate (Xyrem®)—which is approved for the treatment of a sleep disorder called *narcolepsy*—may offer help with pain, fatigue, and sleep disturbances in fibromyalgia. Sodium oxybate gained notoriety as a "date rape" drug; to reduce the risk for abuse, it can only be prescribed using strict prescribing guidelines and a central pharmacy to make sure extra doses are not sold and abused. Large, well-designed clinical trials have found good benefit for symptom reduction, and specialists may prescribe this drug to some people with fibromyalgia.

Pain Medications

Pain medications are notoriously ineffective for reducing fibromyalgia pain. A review published in the *Scandinavian Journal of Rheumatology* found that treatment with analgesic medications provided no better

---

A FIBROMYALGIA MEDICATION PRIMER

First-Line Drugs	Second-Line Drugs	Third-Line Drugs
SNRIs: duloxetine (Cymbalta®) 60 mg once or twice a day and milnacipran (Savella®) 50–100 mg twice a day	Tricyclic antidepressants: amitriptyline (Elavil®) 25 mg at bedtime	SSRIs: fluoxetine (Prozac®) 10–60 mg/day and paroxetine (Paxil®) 20–40 mg/day
Pregabalin (Lyrica®) 450 mg a day	Gabapentin (Neurontin®) 400–800 mg three times daily	
	Tramadol 37.5 mg plus acetaminophen (Ultracet®) 325 mg every 6 hours, as needed	

SNRI, serotonin norepinephrine reuptake inhibitor; SSRI, selective serotonin reuptake inhibitor

pain reduction than treatment with a placebo (or sugar pill). Analgesics, such as acetaminophen and nonsteroidal anti-inflammatory drugs (NSAIDs), as well as strong opioid (narcotic) pain medications, are generally ineffective for reducing fibromyalgia pain. One analgesic medication that *has* been shown to help reduce fibromyalgia pain is a combination of tramadol (Ultram®) 37.5 mg and acetaminophen 325 mg.

SUMMARY

- ▶ Some medications improve certain fibromyalgia symptoms, such as migraine and IBS.
- ▶ Other medications—including some of the antidepressants and neuromodulating therapies—may modestly improve several common fibromyalgia symptoms, including pain, sleep disturbance, and fatigue.
- ▶ Pain medications are generally not effective for reducing fibromyalgia pain.

9

Nutritional Products and Supplements

Two in five women with fibromyalgia take nutritional supplements, and four in five take at least one vitamin or mineral. The most commonly used supplements are omega fatty acids and glucosamine. The most commonly used vitamins and minerals are vitamin C, vitamin E, and magnesium. While vitamin C and magnesium may have a helpful role for fibromyalgia, other nutritional products and supplements have been shown to be more likely to reduce fibromyalgia symptoms. It's important to know which nutritional products and supplements are most likely to help your fibromyalgia. While information on using these therapies is limited, you can use what is known to help identify those vitamins, minerals, and supplements that might be most worthwhile.

VITAMINS

The two vitamins best studied in fibromyalgia are vitamins D and C. Research looking for vitamin D deficiency in fibromyalgia has produced conflicting results. A study published in the *Journal of Clinical Rheumatology* found no increased risk for vitamin D deficiency in people with fibromyalgia, and there was no correlation between vitamin D levels and pain severity. Other studies that tested the effects of vitamin D supplementation produced conflicting results for relief of fibromyalgia symptoms, even among people with documented vitamin D deficiency.

A single small study that treated 12 women with fibromyalgia with vitamin C supplements for 1 month found a reduction in disability with vitamin C that was lost after it was discontinued.

MINERALS

It is unknown whether mineral supplementation might be helpful for fibromyalgia. Research has shown reduced levels of zinc and magnesium in people with fibromyalgia, and low zinc has been correlated with fibromyalgia tender points. Low magnesium has been linked to fatigue. Studies are not available as to whether supplementation with zinc might be beneficial. Combining magnesium with malic acid (the active ingredient in many sour or tart foods) may be beneficial, although no benefits could be documented in well-designed, controlled studies.

HERBS AND SUPPLEMENTS

The most effective supplements for fibromyalgia include S-adenosyl methionine and melatonin, taken at bedtime. S-adenosyl methionine is also called SAMe. This supplement affects a number of brain chemicals important for reducing the symptoms of fibromyalgia, including norepinephrine, dopamine, and serotonin. Research studies show improvements in pain, fatigue, and depression in people with fibromyalgia who use SAMe.

Melatonin is a hormone secreted by the pineal gland in the brain, and it is important for healthy sleep. A recent, well-designed study published in the *Journal of Pineal Research* found that melatonin was as effective as the antidepressant fluoxetine for reducing fibromyalgia

Nutritional Supplement Primer

A number of research studies have tested which supplements are likely to help reduce fibromyalgia symptoms. The treatments shown to help people with fibromyalgia include:

▶ Vitamin C, 500–1,000 mg daily

▶ Vitamin D replacement when blood levels of vitamin D levels are tested as low; vitamin D dose depends on the level of vitamin D deficiency

▶ S-adenosyl methionine, also called SAMe, 800 mg daily

▶ Melatonin, 3 mg taken 30 minutes before bed

▶ Freshwater algae *Chlorella pyrenoidosa*, 10 mg tablet plus 100 mL liquid daily

▶ Coenzyme Q10, 100–200 mg daily

▶ Carnitine, 1,000–1,500 mg daily

▶ Fish oil, 1,500 mg three times daily

Some studies suggest that the following supplements *might* be helpful, but studies in people with fibromyalgia haven't been done yet:

▶ Magnesium

▶ Probiotics for digestive symptoms

▶ Zinc

pain, sleep disturbance, fatigue, and disability. However, fluoxetine is one of the less effective antidepressants for fibromyalgia.

Supplementation with carnitine, chlorella, coenzyme Q10, and omega-3 fatty acids may help reduce some fibromyalgia symptoms.

Always talk to your health care provider before taking any supplement and let her know what supplements you're currently using.

SUMMARY

▶ Vitamin C may reduce fibromyalgia symptoms.
▶ Vitamin D may be helpful if your vitamin D level is low.

▶ Zinc and magnesium levels are often low in people with fibromyalgia. It is not known whether taking these mineral supplements will reduce symptoms.

▶ SAMe and melatonin have both been shown to improve fibromyalgia symptoms.

10

Planning for Pregnancy
When You Have Fibromyalgia

As discussed in Chapter 5, women with fibromyalgia can generally expect to have normal pregnancies, with no increased risk of a miscarriage or pregnancy complications. However, fibromyalgia symptoms can become more of a problem during pregnancy—especially during the last trimester and the first month after delivery.

Pregnancy causes many physical changes. Unfortunately, most women—including those *without* fibromyalgia—experience a number of unpleasant symptoms during pregnancy:

- ▶ Back pain occurs in 81 percent of pregnant women
- ▶ Nausea in 72 percent
- ▶ Extremity or joint pain in 59 percent
- ▶ Stomach or abdominal pain in 57 percent
- ▶ Digestive problems in 50 percent
- ▶ Shortness of breath in 49 percent
- ▶ Headaches in 49 percent

Many of the same pain-reducing techniques used for fibromyalgia may also help reduce pregnancy-related pain and other problems you might develop. Be sure to let your doctor know if you develop any new health concerns during your pregnancy.

Medication options for fibromyalgia are quite limited during pregnancy and nursing. However, the non-drug treatments discussed in Chapters 6 and 7, which are the foundation of managing fibromyalgia, may continue to be used effectively throughout pregnancy and nursing. Developing a treatment program based in non-drug therapies that you can continue during pregnancy is an important first step in pregnancy planning.

Fibromyalgia should not be a barrier to a successful pregnancy. Many other women share your concerns. Pregnancy often creates new challenges as your body changes. You might experience morning sickness, difficulty sleeping, and new aches and pains. Although you may need to modify your treatment regimen, women with fibromyalgia can safely use a variety of effective treatments during pregnancy.

Is Fibromyalgia Keeping You From Having Children?

A study published in the *Clinical Journal of Pain* found that women with fibromyalgia are less likely to have a baby. This study compared the number of children born to women with a painful jaw condition called *temporomandibular dysfunction* (TMD) but no fibromyalgia, women with TMD plus fibromyalgia, and healthy women without pain issues. Women with fibromyalgia had 10 percent fewer pregnancies than either the TMD women without fibromyalgia or the pain-free women. The percentage of women who had never been pregnant was also highest in women with fibromyalgia:

- ▶ 36 percent of the women with fibromyalgia had never been pregnant.
- ▶ 31 percent with TMD but no fibromyalgia had never been pregnant.
- ▶ 27 percent of the healthy women had never been pregnant.

Although having children may be affected by fertility problems, as well as by choice, studies show that women with fibromyalgia have no more menstrual irregularities or difficulty conceiving than other women, even though they are less likely to have children.

If you're having concerns about becoming pregnant, know that you're not alone. Talk to your doctor if you are interested in having a baby and the time seems right, but you're concerned that your fibromyalgia will become unbearable or you won't be able to manage

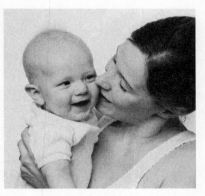

Women with fibromyalgia are less likely to become pregnant.

a baby. Making plans for each stage of pregnancy can help reduce concerns about keeping symptoms under control.

PLANNING FOR PREGNANCY

Be sure to talk to your doctor regularly about your concerns about and plans for adding to your family. If you don't plan to have children, discuss your contraception options. Once you decide it's the right time to become pregnant, schedule an appointment with your doctor to make plans for your future pregnancy.

The pregnancy planning stage is an ideal time to maximize your use of effective non-drug therapies to reduce your fibromyalgia symptoms. You should also review your medications with the doctor who treats your fibromyalgia *and* with your gynecologist. Review all of the prescription and over-the-counter drugs, and nutritional supplements you use. Ask how you should adjust your medication regimen to make sure you're only using drugs that are safe during

Ideally, while you are trying to get pregnant, you should use only medications that will be safe for the baby at the time of conception and during early pregnancy.

Planning for Pregnancy

▶ Discuss your plans for conception and contraception openly with your health care provider.

▶ Make sure you're comfortable using typically effective non-drug techniques:

- Ask about a referral to a behavioral pain psychologist for behavioral therapies, relaxation, and stress management therapy training.

- Ask about working with a fitness trainer or physical therapist to develop an effective aerobic and strength-training exercise program.

- Change your aerobic exercise program to limit jarring activities and exercises that might put you at risk for falling or hitting your abdomen.

- If you take fitness or yoga classes, talk about modifications you may need to make as your pregnancy progresses.

- Consider meeting with a dietician for nutritional assistance if you have significant digestive problems, such as irritable bowel syndrome (IBS).

- Make sure you get sufficient sleep.

▶ Start taking a daily multivitamin containing at least 400 mg of folate.

▶ Review your medications and develop a safe treatment plan you can use while trying to conceive and when pregnant:

- Tell your doctor about any prescription, over-the-counter, and nutritional supplements you are using or considering using.

pregnancy. Ideally, while you are trying to get pregnant, you should use only medications that will be safe for the baby at the time of conception and during early pregnancy.

CHOOSING SAFE DRUGS WHEN YOU'RE PREGNANT

Most women do not want to take any medications during pregnancy. However, *most* women—including those who don't have fibromyalgia—do use medications at some point during pregnancy. A survey of 578 women in the United States found that most of them used prescription, over-the-counter, or nutritional therapies, not including prenatal vitamins, minerals, or iron:

▶ 93 percent of women self-medicated with at least one over-the-counter medication, and 21 percent used five or more over-the-counter medications during pregnancy.

▶ 60 percent used a prescription medication. The most commonly used prescriptions were antibiotics, respiratory drugs, medications for stomach ailments, and narcotics.

▶ 45 percent of the women in the survey used an herbal product.

A survey of over 14,000 pregnancies in the United Kingdom reported that nine in ten women used a prescription, over-the-counter, or nutritional therapy at some point during pregnancy, most commonly analgesics. Analgesics were used by 40 percent of women during the first two trimesters; 31 percent used them during the third trimester.

No drug is 100 percent safe to use with absolutely no side effects or risks. When you're pregnant, your doctor will consider the possible side effects and risks for both you *and* your baby from any medication you might take. Medication options are generally more limited when you're pregnant, because of the possible risks to the baby.

As described in Chapter 8, medications can provide modest symptom reduction for fibromyalgia. Painkillers (analgesics) are generally ineffective and should be avoided. Drugs that are more effective in reducing fibromyalgia symptoms, such as antidepressants and pregabalin, should be avoided during pregnancy unless symptoms are severe and the possible risks are balanced by the potential benefits.

Most women do use drugs at some point during pregnancy, so it's important to talk to your doctor to find out what options are safe.

Be sure to tell the delivery staff at the hospital about any drugs you have been using, so the pediatrician can be prepared to support your baby during and after delivery, if needed.

Antidepressants

Most women who take an antidepressant during pregnancy do not have difficulties with their pregnancy, but they are at increased risk for miscarriage and other complications. Therefore, antidepressants are generally reserved for treating only severe depression during pregnancy.

Antidepressants may be necessary to treat severe mood disorders during pregnancy. They are infrequently recommended during pregnancy, due to the small risk of miscarriage or birth defects with most groups of antidepressants. Problems have been noted with antidepressants during both the early and late stages of pregnancy.

Antidepressants that affect serotonin reuptake—such as the serotonin and norepinephrine reuptake inhibitors typically recommended for fibromyalgia—have been linked to increased risks for miscarriage, low birth weight, and respiratory distress in the baby. These drugs cross the placenta and can also lead to *neonatal behavioral syndrome*, which causes the baby to be jittery, agitated, and experience excessive crying, feeding difficulties, and breathing problems. For these reasons, antidepressants are generally avoided during pregnancy.

Neuromodulating Drugs

Neuromodulating therapies used in fibromyalgia, such as pregabalin and gabapentin, were originally developed to control seizures in people with epilepsy. A 2009 study published in the *New England Journal of Medicine* linked their use during pregnancy with a slight lowering of IQ scores in 3-year-old children who had been exposed to the drugs before birth. The drugs involved—carbamazepine, lamotrigine, phenytoin, and valproate—are not typically used to treat fibromyalgia. The two fibromyalgia drugs that *are* also used to control seizures in some people—pregabalin and gabapentin—were not included in the study.

Information concerning the safety of pregabalin during pregnancy is limited, and this drug is generally avoided unless it's considered medically necessary and the benefits outweigh the potential risks.

More information is available for gabapentin, mostly from small studies of women who used gabapentin to control seizures during pregnancy. In general, it does not seem to be linked to increased risks for miscarriage, low birth weight, or birth defects. Gabapentin may be used in early pregnancy and then discontinued in the third trimester because of possible interference with the baby's bone development.

The neuromodulating drugs topiramate and valproate, antiseizure medications that are sometimes used to prevent migraines, have been linked to serious birth defects, and should be avoided during pregnancy.

Sleep Medications

Limited safety information is available about using either tizanidine or sodium oxybate during pregnancy. In general, these drugs are only used for treating severe symptoms when safer treatments are not feasible and the benefits are believed to outweigh possible risks.

Pain Medications

Analgesics generally do not reduce fibromyalgia pain. Sometimes, however, they are recommended to treat other types of pain that develop during pregnancy. Safe medication options include acetaminophen throughout pregnancy, and nonsteroidal anti-inflammatory drugs (NSAIDs) such as aspirin and ibuprofen during the second trimester. NSAIDs should be avoided while you are trying to get pregnant and during the first trimester because they have been linked to miscarriage. Using NSAIDs during the third trimester can affect the development of the baby's heart, causing premature closure of the *ductus arteriosus*, a shunt that bypasses the lungs and moves blood directly from the baby's heart through the body. This shunt normally closes only after birth.

Premature closure of the ductus arteriosus stresses the heart and breathing system for the developing baby, which can affect development of the heart, blood vessels, and pulmonary system and can result in potentially serious complications.

Narcotics have traditionally been considered to be relatively safe during pregnancy. However, a recent study in the *American Journal of Obstetrics and Gynecology* that included data from the National Birth Defects Prevention Study showed about double the risk for heart

Pain Medications During Pregnancy

▶ Acetaminophen:
  - Generally considered safe to use during pregnancy.
▶ Nonsteroidal anti-inflammatory drugs (aspirin, ibuprofen [Motrin®] and naproxen [Naprosyn®]):
  - Avoid when trying to get pregnant and during early pregnancy, because they can increase your risk for having a miscarriage.
  - Considered a safer pain medication option during the middle of pregnancy.
  - Avoid in the third trimester because these drugs can interfere with the baby's heart development.
▶ Aspirin:
  - Generally avoided during pregnancy.
  - Large studies have shown no increased risk when used during the first trimester, so don't worry too much if you used aspirin before you knew you were pregnant.
▶ Tramadol (Ultram®, Ultracet®):
  - Limited information is available about the safety of tramadol during pregnancy. It is generally avoided unless felt to be medically necessary.
  - Long-term use should be avoided near delivery because tramadol crosses the placenta and withdrawal symptoms can occur in the baby.
▶ Narcotics:
  - Small amounts for limited periods of time can be safe to use during mid to late pregnancy; however, narcotics generally do not reduce fibromyalgia pain.

defects, a digestive disorder, and spina bifida when narcotics were used during the month before pregnancy or during the first trimester.

Treating Nausea or "Morning Sickness"

During the first weeks of pregnancy, nausea or "morning sickness" can be particularly difficult. Ask your doctor about how to best manage morning sickness when you are developing your pregnancy treatment plan. Both lifestyle changes and nutritional therapies are often helpful.

The American College of Obstetricians and Gynecologists (ACOG) recommends treating pregnancy-related nausea with vitamin B_6 and ginger, both of which are safe and effective. In one study, pregnant women used either ginger or vitamin B_6 over a 4-day period to treat nausea. Nausea severity decreased by about 20 percent with either treatment after the first day of treatment. After 4 days, nausea had decreased by over half with ginger and by one-third with vitamin B_6.

Managing Nausea During Pregnancy

▶ Drink small amounts of cold, clear, carbonated drinks between meals. Try ginger ale or lemon-lime soda, clear broth, juice diluted with water, gelatin, electrolyte drinks such as Gatorade and Pedialyte, and popsicles.

▶ Eat in a cool room with good ventilation.

▶ If odors increase nausea, don't eat in or near the kitchen, and try frozen or prepared foods to reduce cooking odors.

▶ Slowly eat small portions of easily tolerated foods such as bananas, applesauce, rice, and toast.

▶ An empty stomach can aggravate nausea. Keep a tin of crackers by your bedside to eat if you wake up during the night. Eat a few crackers before getting up in the morning. Eat frequent, small meals and healthy snacks throughout the day.

▶ Add eggs and yogurt to your diet as good sources of protein and nutrition.

▶ Choose salty foods instead of sweets.

▶ Avoid spicy, fried, or fatty foods.

Talk to your doctor about treating mild nausea with 1 gram of ginger or 30 mg of vitamin B₆ daily for up to 3–4 days. Both treatments are safe, effective, and recommended by the American College of Obstetricians and Gynecologists.

Another herbal therapy, An-Tai-Yin, has been used to treat morning sickness. However, it has been linked to increased risk for birth defects when used during the first trimester and should *not* be used when you are trying to get pregnant or during early pregnancy.

Applying acupressure over the wrist at the P6 acupressure point can also relieve nausea. This acupressure point is located between the tendons about two to three finger widths above your wrist crease. Make firm, deep circular motions over this area for several minutes to reduce nausea.

If your nausea is severe, talk to your doctor about possible prescription medications. The nausea drug ondansetron (Zofran®) is considered relatively safe during pregnancy, and obstetricians often prescribe promethazine (Phenergan®).

TAKE ADVANTAGE OF SAFE, EFFECTIVE NON-DRUG THERAPIES

Pain and fatigue often become worse during pregnancy, so it's important to get your symptoms under the best control possible *before* you become pregnant. This is a great time to make sure you're taking advantage of effective non-drug treatments, such as exercise, strength training, and behavioral ther-

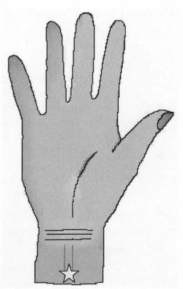

The P6 acupressure point for nausea (star). Reproduced with the permission of Marcus and Bain. *The Woman's Migraine Toolkit.* Diamedica Publishing: New York, NY;2011, page 157.

First Trimester
from conception to week 14

Second Trimester
from week 15 to week 27

Third Trimester
from week 28 to delivery

Pregnancy is divided into three trimesters starting from the time of conception and ending with delivery after approximately 36–40 weeks of pregnancy.

apies. These are great techniques to use when you're trying to get pregnant and throughout pregnancy. If you are already trained in these techniques, consider scheduling an appointment with a therapist for booster sessions to help reinforce and improve your skills.

Exercising When You're Pregnant

The ACOG recommends aerobic exercise, strength training, and flexibility exercises during pregnancy unless you have medical conditions that prevent you from exercising, such as a complicated pregnancy or significant heart or lung disease. Strength training should generally be limited to using only light weights. You should also limit isometric exercises when you're pregnant.

A recent review of exercise during pregnancy in the journal Physical Medicine & Rehabilitation *found that healthy women could safely exercise up to 60 minutes or more per day during pregnancy. Aerobics, using a stationary bike or StairMaster, and strength training, are all considered safe forms of exercise.*

The ACOG recommends a daily total of 30 minutes of aerobic exercise for healthy pregnant women. They provide free educational pamphlets on exercise and fitness during pregnancy at their website (see Chapter 13).

Aerobic exercise during pregnancy can be good for you *and* your baby. Women who exercise during pregnancy are less likely to develop preeclampsia and pregnancy-related diabetes. Aerobic exercise often needs to be modified during pregnancy:

▶ Most women can continue to exercise throughout pregnancy, although adjustments may be needed.

▶ Talk to your doctor before starting a new aerobic exercise program.

▶ Reduce high-impact exercise. Consider walking, low-impact or water aerobics, swimming, or riding a stationary bike.

▶ Avoid activities that might put you at risk for falling or trauma, including contact sports, soccer, basketball, gymnastics, skiing, horseback riding, and tennis or racquetball. Also avoid scuba diving.

▶ Limit exercises done while lying flat on your back.

▶ Stop exercising and contact your doctor right away if you have severe abdominal pain, problems with breathing, dizziness, or blurred vision, or vaginal fluid drainage during or after exercise.

How Much Should I Exercise When I'm Pregnant?

▶ Talk to your doctor about any exercise restrictions you may have.

▶ Start low and go slow. If you have been inactive before becoming pregnant, take your time getting to the target of 30 minutes per day.

▶ Limit individual exercise sessions to a maximum of 30 minutes.

▶ Ideally, do several 10–15 minute exercise sessions throughout the day, rather than a single longer session.

▶ The ACOG cautions that pregnancy is not a good time to improve your level of physical fitness, especially if you were reasonably active before pregnancy, in which case you can expect your overall fitness and activity level to drop somewhat as you go through pregnancy.

A large survey of women collected through the Danish National Birth Cohort showed that swimming in a pool is safe during pregnancy. The women who swam during pregnancy actually had slightly lower risks of experiencing preterm labor or having a baby with a birth defect, compared to those who didn't exercise. Another study conducted with this same group of women found that women who were less health conscious, smoked, or considered their health to be normal or less than normal were less likely to exercise during pregnancy, so some of the benefits seen with swimming may be attributed to the fact that healthier women are more likely to exercise. On the other hand, this study does support that swimming is safe during pregnancy.

Healthy women with fibromyalgia can usually continue low-impact aerobics and modest strength training during pregnancy.

Modest strength training can also continue during pregnancy for most healthy women. In one study, 160 sedentary pregnant women were randomly assigned to exercise three times weekly for 35–40 minutes per session or to continue not exercising. Light resistance and toning exercises performed during the second and third trimesters did not affect labor and delivery, birth weight, or overall newborn health. The researchers noted that "women in the training group were rather pleased with the exercise training, and all of the women reported their intention to be physically active in future pregnancies."

Stay Hydrated

▶ The average woman needs to drink 2–3 liters (8–10 eight-ounce glasses) of water every day.

▶ Pregnant women generally need to drink an additional half-liter of water each day.

▶ Keep 1-liter bottles of water in the refrigerator to make sure you're drinking enough each day.

▶ Drink an extra glass of water before and after exercise sessions.

When you're pregnant, you need to be careful about hydration, nutrition, and temperature regulation. Make sure you drink extra water throughout the day, and before and after exercise, to stay hydrated. Also limit the duration of each exercise session to avoid problems with energy balance or overheating.

Sleep

Sleep problems tend to be aggravated by pregnancy. A study in *Sleep Medicine* monitored sleep patterns in 325 women before pregnancy and

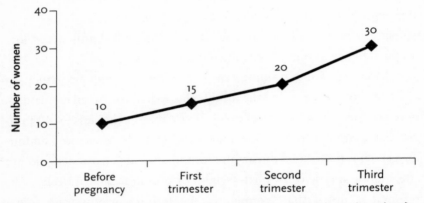

Among 100 pregnant women, how many can expect to experience restless sleep?

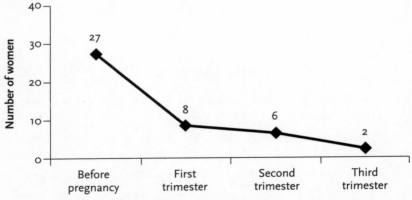

Among 100 pregnant women, how many can expect to sleep straight through the night without wake-ups?

during each trimester. Sleep became more disrupted and less restful as pregnancy progressed, showing that most women have problems with sleep during pregnancy. You may find sleep more of a problem if you also have fibromyalgia. Healthy sleep habits (see Chapter 7) are particularly important when you're pregnant, so be sure to practice them before you get pregnant.

Acupuncture and Acupressure for Sleep Management

Although acupuncture does not generally reduce fibromyalgia symptoms, acupuncture using specific points on the ear—called *auricular* acupuncture—may improve both sleep quality and total amount of sleep time. The *auricle* is the medical term for the part of your ear that you can see. A small study published in the journal *Acupuncture in Medicine* found acupuncture helpful for reducing insomnia in women during pregnancy. Pregnancy is a good time to try acupuncture as a safe sleep aid.

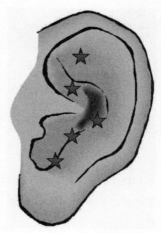

Massaging acupressure points on the ear (stars) for 1 minute before going to bed can improve sleep quality and increase total hours of sleep.

Acupressure has also been shown to improve sleep in older women, although studies have not been conducted in younger women during pregnancy.

Massage

Consider adding massage to your treatment program when you're pregnant. This soothing therapy provides modest benefits for fibromyalgia and is best used along with other effective non-drug treatments, such as exercise and behavioral therapies (see Chapters 6 and 7). Studies sug-

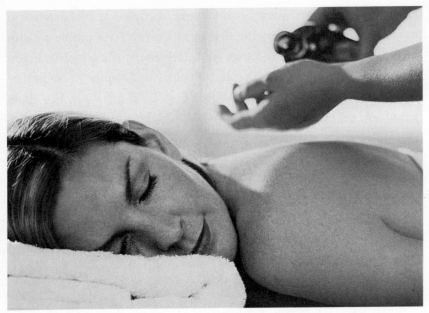

Consider adding massage once or twice a week to your fibromyalgia treatment program when you're pregnant.

gest that once- or twice-weekly massage therapy is optimal for pregnant women with fibromyalgia.

PLANNING YOUR DELIVERY

Try to arrange for labor to occur in a quiet, calm environment to avoid unnecessary stimulation. Talk to the nurses to make sure you can try to walk and change positions frequently during labor when this is feasible, and ask them to provide heat and counter-pressure therapy for your lower back. Plan to use relaxation techniques during labor.

Knowing that your symptoms may flare during the end of pregnancy and during the first few weeks after the baby's born shouldn't stop you from having a baby. However, you may need extra support to make the arrival of your baby as enjoyable as possible.

Planning for the End of Pregnancy and Delivery

▶ Talk to your doctor at the beginning of pregnancy about treatments and techniques that you can use during the end of pregnancy and after delivery to help reduce flares.

▶ Use non-drug treatments regularly, even when your symptoms are modest (see Chapters 6 and 7).

▶ Arrange for others to take over household chores toward the end of your pregnancy and after delivery. This doesn't mean you need to find someone else to care for baby, but it can be helpful to have someone assist with cleaning, shopping, and laundry so you can enjoy and bond with your new baby.

▶ Make plans for contraception after delivery, such as condoms, spermicides, and/or an intrauterine device. Estrogen-containing contraceptives are generally not permitted right after delivery, but progestin-only preparations may be used.

Will I Be Able to Nurse My Baby?

The American Academy of Pediatrics recommends that new mothers *exclusively* breastfeed their babies for the first 6 months, with nursing continuing for at least the baby's first year of life. Although breastfeeding may be ideal, most mothers only nurse during the first few days of a baby's life, and only two in five are still breastfeeding when the baby is 6 months old. Most doctors agree that any breastfeeding is good, and that more breastfeeding is better.

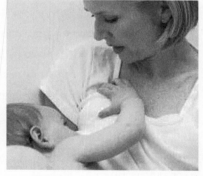

Although nursing does not aggravate symptoms for most women, breastfeeding can be challenging for new mothers with fibromyalgia. In a study of nine

Breastfeeding provides important nutrients and immune factors to your baby. It can also help you bond with your baby and lose pregnancy weight faster. Women who breastfeed have lower risks for developing breast and ovarian cancers and rheumatoid arthritis.

women with fibromyalgia, all were frustrated by the nursing experience, describing similar issues that negatively affected breastfeeding, including:

- ▶ Muscle pain:
  - Problems finding a comfortable position for nursing
  - Stiffness after staying in one position too long
- ▶ Fatigue can interfere with nursing, caring for the baby, caring for older children, keeping up with household chores.
- ▶ Medications were limited when nursing.
- ▶ Concerns that their milk supply wasn't enough or that nursing took too much time
- ▶ Guilt over having to stop nursing earlier than originally planned

Making plans to frequently change positions during nursing and enlisting others to help with household chores may improve your ability to continue nursing. Remember that your baby benefits from *any* time spent nursing, so don't worry if you're not able to continue for as long as you might like.

What Drugs Can I Safely Use While Nursing?

Safe pain medications when you're breastfeeding include acetaminophen, ibuprofen, and naproxen. Low-dose narcotics are safe as a one-time treatment, but repeated use should be avoided because they can build up in some babies. As already discussed, these analgesics have limited benefit for reducing fibromyalgia pain. Tramadol may be more effective for fibromyalgia pain; however, it should be avoided when nursing, because it gets into the breast milk and its possible effects on the baby are not known.

The Academy of Breastfeeding Medicine Protocol Committee recommends that nursing mothers use antidepressants if they have moderate or severe depression. Antidepressants are generally avoided for treating other conditions, such as chronic pain, when breastfeeding

Tips for Successful Nursing

► At the beginning of the third trimester:

- Talk to your doctor about your fibromyalgia treatment program after the baby is born.

- Set up realistic expectations for nursing.

- Consider adding booster sessions with exercise and behavioral therapists for non-drug pain management skills.

- Consider meeting with a lactation counselor.

- Tell your doctor if you notice problems with your mood.

► Before delivery:

- Talk to your family about prioritizing and scheduling essential chores for the baby and the family after delivery. Delegate chores to others.

- Make sure you eat well and stay hydrated by drinking enough water.

- Talk to your doctor about what to expect in terms of increased fatigue after delivery.

- Tell your doctor if you are noticing problems with your mood.

- Review your fibromyalgia treatment plan for after delivery with your doctor.

► Before leaving the hospital after delivery:

- Get advice from the nurses about breastfeeding your baby. Let your health care team know about any difficulties or concerns you might have for when you get home.

► Remember that your baby receives important health benefits from breast-feeding, even if you're not able to nurse as long as you might like.

► Remember to find comfortable positions when nursing, such as nursing lying on your side or using a pillow or sling to help support the weight of the baby.

► Remember to change positions frequently during nursing sessions to reduce getting sore and stiff.

► Plan to nurse at home in a quiet, comfortable environment.

► If you have a lactation counselor, get in touch with her to review your concerns.

► Review your treatment plan for fibromyalgia symptoms with your doctor. Make sure you know what to do when symptoms flare.

► Schedule a follow-up visit with your doctor for soon after hospital discharge to reassess your fibromyalgia treatments.

because the long-term effects of antidepressants on the baby's developing nervous system are unknown.

Gabapentin also gets into breast milk, although the blood levels are low in nursing babies drinking breast milk from mothers treated with the drug, and problems with these babies have not been seen. Otherwise, there is limited information about the effects of gabapentin and pregabalin with nursing, so these are also generally avoided. Likewise, there is limited information about the use of sodium oxybate when nursing, so this should similarly be avoided.

Exercising After Delivery

You can start exercising as soon after delivery as you're physically able to do so. Remember that your body goes through many changes during pregnancy, and that these changes last for several weeks after your baby is born. You will also likely experience increased fibromyalgia pain and fatigue after delivery. So plan for a gradual return to the activities you were doing before you became pregnant.

If you are breastfeeding, try nursing before exercising to avoid discomfort from exercising with engorged breasts. When you're nursing, drink one glass of water with each meal *plus* a glass of water every time you nurse your baby. You should also drink extra water before and after exercise to stay hydrated.

CAN I USE NATURAL THERAPIES WHEN I'M PREGNANT OR NURSING?

Standard doses of vitamins and minerals are generally safe during pregnancy and nursing. It's important to get enough vitamins and minerals for your health and the health of your baby. Most pregnant women are prescribed a prenatal vitamin that includes a wide range of vitamins and minerals, including at least 400 mg of folate. Always talk to your

NUTRITIONAL SUPPLEMENTS FOR FIBROMYALGIA DURING PREGNANCY AND BREASTFEEDING

Safety Rating	Pregnancy	Breastfeeding
Safe	*Chlorella pyrenoidosa*	Fish oil; limit dose to no more than 3 grams daily
	Fish oil made from fish bodies; avoid products made from fish liver (like cod liver oil) and products with high-dose omega-3 fatty acids; limit dose to 3 grams daily or less*	Magnesium**
		Probiotics *Lactobacillus* and *Bifidobacterium*
		Vitamin C and D**
	Ginger for nausea	Zinc**
	Magnesium**	
	Probiotics *Lactobacillus* and *Bifidobacterium*	
	Vitamin C and D**	
	Zinc**	
Avoid because information is not known or they are unsafe	Carnitine	Carnitine
	Coenzyme Q10	*Chlorella pyrenoidosa*
	Melatonin	Coenzyme Q10
	Probiotic *Saccharomyces*	Melatonin
	S-adenosyl methionine (SAMe)	Probiotic *Saccharomyces*
		S-adenosyl methionine (SAMe)

*Fish oil may need to be avoided if you have bleeding problems. Always talk to your doctor before taking fish oil to make sure it's safe for you.

**Do not take extra vitamins or minerals without first checking with your doctor. You will likely be prescribed prenatal vitamins when pregnant and nursing.

doctor before taking any additional vitamin or mineral supplements, to make sure that you don't take too high a dose that might cause problems for you or the baby.

Several nutritional supplements used to treat fibromyalgia have been studied for safety and possible beneficial effects during pregnancy.

The probiotics *Lactobacillus* and *Bifidobacterium* have been shown to be safe during pregnancy and for 3 months after delivery during breastfeeding. One interesting study treated women with either probiotics or a placebo (sugar pill) during the end of pregnancy and for the first 3 months while nursing. When the children were 2 years old, the researchers evaluated the 138 children who had been exposed to probiotics and the 140 who had not. Interestingly, children whose mothers took probiotics at the end of pregnancy and when nursing were half as likely to have an itchy skin condition resembling eczema called *atopic dermatitis*. Another study, published in the *Journal of Medicinal Food*, showed that babies whose mothers had taken 6 grams of *Chlorella pyrenoidosa* tablets during the last 6 months of pregnancy had lower concentrations of environmental toxins and higher concentrations of healthy antibodies.

Always talk to your doctor before taking nutritional supplements when you are pregnant or nursing.

Always talk to your doctor before taking nutritional supplements when you're pregnant or nursing.

SUMMARY

▶ Fibromyalgia symptoms tend to worsen with pregnancy, especially at the end of pregnancy and after the baby is born.

▶ Nursing should not aggravate overall fibromyalgia symptoms, but it can provide unique challenges for new mothers with fibromyalgia; these usually can be addressed by adjusting nursing positions and delegating some household chores to others.

▶ Develop a strong base of effective non-drug treatments before becoming pregnant, and plan to use them regularly throughout pregnancy and when breastfeeding.

▶ Medications are generally limited during pregnancy and nursing.

▶ Several nutritional therapies can be safely used during pregnancy and nursing.

▶ Additional therapies to help reduce fibromyalgia symptoms during pregnancy include massage, acupuncture, and acupressure.

Part IV

Putting Knowledge Into Practice

Most fibromyalgia treatments do not produce an immediate improvement in symptoms, but you should be able to get a sense of whether they are starting to be helpful after using them consistently for 2–3 months. At that point, you must decide if you want to keep using the same treatments, add additional therapies, or switch to something entirely new.

It can be difficult to judge whether your symptoms are improving, because most fibromyalgia treatments provide only modest improvements rather than dramatic results. It's hard to remember how you felt 2–3 months before you started a treatment, because some days and weeks will be worse than others. You don't want to persevere with treatments that aren't helping, but you also don't want to abandon therapies that have started to provide some improvement—even when that initial improvement might be small.

Using tools to systematically monitor your symptoms is an effective approach to monitoring your progress. Diaries to log your treatments are also important motivational tools to help keep you on track. Evaluating these tools with your doctor can provide a clearer picture of what's working, what's not, and what changes might be helpful.

Your doctor is one of your best resources for better understanding your fibromyalgia and what you can do to relieve your symptoms. Learning to be an effective communicator by sharing information you've collected in diaries, bringing short lists of important issues to address at appointments, and learning to discuss your concerns openly can be important first steps toward successful fibromyalgia management. Other reliable resources include websites that provide the latest information.

Measuring Success

Using diaries to track your most troublesome symptoms is a useful way to look for symptom patterns and changes in them as you try different treatments. They can help you notice even modest improvements that you might miss otherwise, and share what has happened between visits with your health care providers. It's important to remember that diaries, like most things in life, can be overdone. Simply tracking your symptoms day after day for prolonged periods of time can become tedious and disheartening, and might even make some symptoms worse by focusing on them too much.

The two best times to track your symptoms are before a new doctor visit and after you have started a new treatment. Completing a diary once a week for a few weeks, or for 1 week each month for a few months, can provide information about whether your symptoms are improving or not.

Exercise diaries can be great motivational tools to remind you to keep up your aerobic exercise and relaxation sessions. Again, you don't need to complete these diaries day after day indefinitely. Instead, use them until exercise and relaxation have become a regular part of your routine.

When you're working with a health care provider, it's also important to remember that every clinician has his own methods for monitoring progress and tracking symptoms. Some will ask to review your diaries; others might prefer a verbal report about your progress. Some of the tools in this chapter require calculations to obtain scores, and many doctors would rather spend office visit time talking with you, rather than making calculations. Your doctor may also become concerned that you're spending too much time logging symptoms and not enough time making important healthy lifestyle changes. As a result, she may suggest that you take a break from recording your symptoms. Physicians usually recommend methods they have found to be most successful, so it's important to stay open to your own health care provider's directions on how to best track your progress.

TRACK YOUR SYMPTOMS

Monitoring symptoms can provide helpful information to you and your health care provider, and identify your most troublesome problem areas. Completing your symptom logs before visiting the doctor and bringing the results with you will help you to more effectively communicate with him. It also means you won't leave your appointment thinking, "Drat. I forgot to tell him about . . . . "

Once you have started a treatment program, complete the logs every week or so to help monitor your progress. Most fibromyalgia treatments take several weeks to produce noticeable effects. Sometimes, it's hard to recognize that you're making progress, especially when improvements occur gradually. Being able to go back several weeks to review your symptoms before treatment can help you decide if your treatment is helping or not. Being able to identify improvements can prevent you from abandoning treatments that might have become more beneficial if you had continued them.

Pain, Sleep, and Fatigue

The *FibroFatigue Scale* was developed by researchers in Sweden. This tool can be used to rate a wide range of common fibromyalgia symp-

A MODIFIED FIBROFATIGUE SCALE

Fibromyalgia Symptom	Rate Symptom Severity 0 = no or minimal symptoms 6 = severe and disabling symptoms						
	0	1	2	3	4	5	6
Aches and pains							
Muscular tension							
Fatigue							
Concentration difficulties							
Failing memory							
Irritability							
Sadness							
Sleep disturbances							
Autonomic disturbances, such as heart fluttering or palpitations, difficulty breathing, dizziness, excess sweating, cold hands and feet, dry mouth, or frequent urination							
Irritable bowel, including abdominal pain, diarrhea, constipation, or bloating							
Headache							
Symptoms of infection, including fever, chills, sore throat, or tender lymph nodes							
Other:							
Other:							
Other:							

Circle the symptom that causes you the most trouble.

Write down today's date: _____/_____/_____

Adapted from Zachrisson, et al. *J Psychosom Res.* 2002;52:501–9.

toms. It is a reliable and accurate tool for measuring the severity of fibromyalgia symptoms and changes in symptoms with treatment.

Another tool you can use to keep track of the severity of your symptoms is a simple 0 to 10 scale. This can be used for pain (0 equals

FIBROMYALGIA SYMPTOM SEVERITY LOG

This fibromyalgia symptom severity log lets you log your symptoms in Week 1 before treatment and for 4 weeks after starting treatment (Weeks 2 through 5). Many treatments take several weeks before you can expect to see benefit.

Weekly Log

(Record the date for the first day of each week in boxes below.)

Fibromyalgia Symptom	Week 1	Week 2	Week 3	Week 4	Week 5
Average pain severity (0 = no pain, 10 = excruciating and disabling pain)					
Average number of hours of nighttime sleep (healthy sleep in adults = 7–9 hours nightly)					
Sleep Quality Scale over last 24 hours (0 = best sleep, 10 = worst sleep)					

Add a check for each of the following symptoms that are problematic each week. Add notations to each box to expand, if helpful.

Disability for work or household chores					
Disability for leisure, family, or social activities					
Sleep disturbance					
Bowel problems					
Troublesome headaches					
Excess weight					
Depression or anxiety					

no pain and 10 equals unbearable pain), sleep disturbance (0 when sleep is good and 10 when it is severely disrupted), and fatigue (0 represents no fatigue and 10 the worst fatigue possible). Noting symptoms that are still a problem for you and adding details about the limitations they

---

INSOMNIA SEVERITY INDEX

Rate your sleep over the last 2 weeks:

1. How much difficulty do you have **falling asleep**?

None (0)　　Mild (1)　　Moderate (2)　　Severe (3)　　Very severe (4)

2. How much difficulty do you have **staying asleep**?

None (0)　　Mild (1)　　Moderate (2)　　Severe (3)　　Very severe (4)

3. How much of a problem do you have **waking up too early**?

None (0)　　Mild (1)　　Moderate (2)　　Severe (3)　　Very severe (4)

4. How **satisfied are you** with your current sleeping pattern?

Very satisfied (0)　　Satisfied (1)　　Moderately satisfied (2)
Dissatisfied (3)　　Very dissatisfied (4)

5. How much do **others notice** your sleep impairs your quality of life?

Not notice at all (0)　　Notice a little (1)　　Notice somewhat (2)
Notice much (3)　　Notice very much (4)

6. How **worried or distressed** are you about your sleep?

Not worried at all (0)　　A little worried (1)　　Somewhat worried (2)
Much worried (3)　　Very much worried (4)

7. How much does your sleep **interfere with your daily functioning**?

Not interfering at all (0)　　Interferes a little (1)　　Interferes somewhat (2)
Interferes much (3)　　Interferes very much (4)

Add the scores for each question together to get a possible score from zero to 28. Scores higher than 14 represent moderately severe insomnia. Scores over 21 represent severe insomnia.

Write down today's date: _____/_____/_____

Adapted from Bastien, et al. Validation of the Insomnia Severity Index as an outcome measure for insomnia research. *Sleep Med.* 2001;2:297–307.

impose can help you and your health care provider target treatments. Sleep disturbance also can be measured using the Insomnia Severity Index.

SCREENING FOR DEPRESSION

Name:_____   Date:_____/_____/_____

Please rate each statement, considering how you have been feeling in the last 2–3 days compared with how you normally feel:

	Not True Score = 0	Slightly True Score = 1	Moderately True Score = 2	Very True Score = 3
I find myself stewing over things.				
I feel more vulnerable than usual.				
I am critical of or hard on myself.				
I feel guilty.				
Nothing seems to cheer me up.				
I feel like I've lost my core, or essence.				
I feel depressed.				
I feel less worthwhile.				
I feel hopeless or helpless.				
I feel distant from other people.				

Scoring: Total your scores from each question. A total score of 9 or greater suggests that you may be experiencing depression.

Adapted from Parker G, Hilton T, Bains J, Hadzi-Pavlovic D. Cognitive-based measures screening for depression in the medically ill: The DMI-10 and the DMI-18. *Acta Psychiatr Scand*. 2002;105:419–26. Reprinted from Marcus DA. *Chronic Pain. A Primary Care Guide to Practical Management*. Totowa, NJ: Humana Press, 2009.

Mood

As mentioned in Chapter 1, approximately two in three women with fibromyalgia have difficulty with mood, including depression and anxiety. Periodically completing screening tools for depression and anxiety can help make sure mood disorders are not becoming a problem.

SCREENING FOR ANXIETY

Name:_____ Date:_____/_____/_____

Choose the one description for each item that best describes **how many days** you have been bothered by each of the following over the past **2 weeks**:

	None Score = 0	Several Score = 1	7 or More Score = 2	Nearly Every Day Score = 3
Feeling nervous, anxious, or on edge				
Unable to stop worrying				
Worrying too much about different things				
Problems relaxing				
Feeling restless or unable to sit still				
Feeling irritable or easily annoyed				
Being afraid that something awful might happen				

Scoring: Sum scores from each question. A total score of 5–9 suggests mild anxiety; a score over 10 suggests moderate-severe anxiety.

Adapted from Spitzer RL, Kroenke K, Williams JW, Löwe B. A brief measure for assessing generalized anxiety disorder. The GAD-7. *Arch Intern Med.* 2006;166:1092–7. Reprinted from Marcus DA. *Chronic Pain. A Primary Care Guide to Practical Management.* Totowa, NJ: Humana Press, 2009.

Disability

The Fibromyalgia Impact Questionnaire Revised (FIQR) is a comprehensive assessment of how fibromyalgia may be affecting your life. Fill out this questionnaire and take it to your doctor's appointment to show her how your life is affected by fibromyalgia.

FIBROMYALGIA IMPACT QUESTIONNAIRE REVISED [FIQR]

Name:_____   Date:_____/_____/_____

Question 1. Circle how difficult it has been to do each of the following tasks over the past week from 0 (no difficulty) to 10 (very difficult):

Brush or comb your hair	0 1 2 3 4 5 6 7 8 9 10
Walk continuously for 20 minutes	0 1 2 3 4 5 6 7 8 9 10
Prepare a homemade meal	0 1 2 3 4 5 6 7 8 9 10
Vacuum, scrub, or sweep floors	0 1 2 3 4 5 6 7 8 9 10
Lift and carry a full bag of groceries	0 1 2 3 4 5 6 7 8 9 10
Climb one flight of stairs	0 1 2 3 4 5 6 7 8 9 10
Change bedding	0 1 2 3 4 5 6 7 8 9 10
Sit in a chair for 45 minutes	0 1 2 3 4 5 6 7 8 9 10
Shop for groceries	0 1 2 3 4 5 6 7 8 9 10

Question 2. Rate the overall impact fibromyalgia has had on your life over the last week from 0 (never) to 10 (always):

Fibromyalgia prevented me from accomplishing what I wanted to do this week.	0 1 2 3 4 5 6 7 8 9 10
I was completely overwhelmed by fibromyalgia this week.	0 1 2 3 4 5 6 7 8 9 10

Question 3. Rate the intensity of these fibromyalgia symptoms over the past week from 0 (none) to 10 (very severe).

Pain	0 1 2 3 4 5 6 7 8 9 10
Stiffness	0 1 2 3 4 5 6 7 8 9 10
Depression	0 1 2 3 4 5 6 7 8 9 10
Anxiety	0 1 2 3 4 5 6 7 8 9 10
Tenderness to touch	0 1 2 3 4 5 6 7 8 9 10

| Balance problems | 0 1 2 3 4 5 6 7 8 9 10 |
| Sensitivity to loud noise, bright lights, odors, and cold | 0 1 2 3 4 5 6 7 8 9 10 |

Question 4. Rate the following over the past week from 0 (not a problem) to 10 (quite severe).

Energy level	0 1 2 3 4 5 6 7 8 9 10
Sleep quality	0 1 2 3 4 5 6 7 8 9 10
Memory	0 1 2 3 4 5 6 7 8 9 10

Scoring the FIQR:

1. Add each selected rating for all items in Question 1 and divide by 3.

2. Add ratings for both items in Question 2.

3. Add ratings for all items in Questions 3 and 4; divide total by 2.

4. Add these three scores together for the total FIQR score. Maximum total score = 100. Average score in fibromyalgia patients = 50. Scores over 70 represent severe impact.

Adapted from Bennett RM, Friend R, Jones KD, et al. The Revised Fibromyalgia Impact Questionnaire (FIQR): Validation and psychometric properties. *Arthritis Res Ther.* 2009;11:R120.

Track Your Treatments

Keeping a diary to track your progress can help you continue following your treatment program. Diaries are also helpful for guiding you in progressing at an appropriate pace—not advancing too quickly or too slowly. Be sure to talk with your health care provider if you are not able to advance your program or continue following it, because your program may need to be modified.

Aerobic Exercise Logs

Check the box that corresponds to your level of exercise each day. Your target should be to do at least 20 minutes of aerobic exercise at least 3 days each week. Don't miss too many exercise days, and make sure you

WEEKLY WALKING LOG

	Sunday	Monday	Tuesday	Wednesday	Thursday	Friday	Saturday
1 mile							
1/2 mile							
1/4 mile							
1/8 mile							
Strength training							

WEEKLY BIKING OR SWIMMING LOG

	Sunday	Monday	Tuesday	Wednesday	Thursday	Friday	Saturday
20 minutes							
15 minutes							
10 minutes							
5 minutes							
Strength training							

gradually increase your level of exercise. Also, try to do strength training 2–3 days each week. You can use small weights at the gym or from your sporting goods store, or use small soup or fruit cans for hand weights. More repetitions with smaller weights will be more beneficial than doing only a few repetitions with heavier ones.

Relaxation Log

When you are first learning relaxation techniques, practice them twice daily for 15–20 minutes each. Practice in a quiet environment, and record the actual time you spent in each session. Rate and log tension as none (0), mild (1), moderate (2), or severe (3).

RELAXATION LOG

	Morning Relaxation			Evening Relaxation		
	Time (Minutes)	Tension Before	Tension After	Time (Minutes)	Tension Before	Tension After
Sunday						
Monday						
Tuesday						
Wednesday						
Thursday						
Friday						
Saturday						

UNDERSTANDING MEANINGFUL IMPROVEMENT: HOW DO I KNOW MY TREATMENT IS WORKING?

To determine whether your treatments are helpful, you first have to define what *helpful* means. Everyone wants treatment that relieves all of their symptoms—they'd like a cure. Unfortunately, that's not realistic. *Clinically meaningful improvement* is the amount of relief a person with fibromyalgia needs to experience before she believes that she is benefitting from a treatment plan.

In general, pain needs to improve by approximately 30 percent before the change is considered meaningful. On a 0–10 pain-rating scale—on which 0 equals no pain and 10 equals unbearable pain—your pain would need to decrease by approximately 3 points. Your pain will not be completely gone with this level of change, but it might represent a decrease from severe to moderate.

A decrease in pain severity by 2–3 points on a 0–10-point severity scale indicates that the treatment plan is beneficial.

Researchers from Oregon Health & Science University evaluated the FIQR to determine how much of a change represents meaningful improvement. They found that a decrease of 14 percent was needed to be meaningful. For example, if your FIQR score was 65 before treatment, a drop of 9 points (to a score of 56) would be a 14 percent improvement. This is a more moderate, and noticeable, impact on fibromyalgia.

Sleep studies sometimes define clinically meaningful insomnia as taking at least 30 minutes to get to sleep, waking up for more than 30 minutes during the night, or waking up in the morning at least 60 minutes earlier than planned. A clinically meaningful improvement would be no longer meeting these conditions. Clinically meaningful improvement has also been defined when using the Insomnia Severity Index. In general, a 6-point reduction in the Insomnia Severity Index is considered clinically meaningful.

If you rate your fatigue (weariness, tiredness) over the past week on a scale from 0 (no fatigue) to 10 (fatigue as bad as you can imagine), a decrease of at least 1 point is considered clinically meaningful.

SUMMARY

▶ Tools are available to quantify the severity of a variety of common fibromyalgia symptoms.
▶ Some tools monitor a range of symptoms; others target particular problem areas.
▶ Symptom severity measures can help you communicate better with your health care provider.
▶ Following the results of symptom severity measures can help you determine whether beneficial improvements have occurred.
▶ Clinically meaningful improvements are important treatment outcome targets.

12

Talking to Your Doctor About Fibromyalgia

Peeople with fibromyalgia have two problems that can make a conversation with their physicians difficult: first, most doctor visits are short; and second, your doctor may not understand how disabling fibromyalgia can be. Organizing the time you have with your doctor and helping him by prioritizing the issues you want to discuss during each visit can make your time together more productive.

If you feel as if your doctor is rushing you through your appointment and out the door, you're not alone. The average doctor's visit now lasts only about 20 minutes. While this may be enough time to review how to manage blood pressure, it's probably too short to handle several health issues adequately. If you try to talk about pain, poor sleep, and bowel issues, your doctor will probably become a bit uncomfortable, knowing there's not enough time to cover everything. It's not just the American system that's to blame—the average doctor visit in Europe lasts 10 minutes, and in Japan, only 6 minutes.

The average primary care doctor visit in the United States lasts approximately 20 minutes.

Do most physicians consider fibromyalgia a significant medical condition? When you try to talk to your doctor about your symptoms, do you get the sense that he's really not listening and would rather hear about something else? This reaction is not just because of you—and

219

unfortunately it's *not* unique to your doctor. In a recent study, doctors were asked to rank the status they gave to 38 common medical conditions, including fibromyalgia, based on the standing they believed that each held among doctors. The health issues awarded the highest status included myocardial infarction (heart attack), leukemia, spleen rupture, brain tumor, pulmonary embolism, testicular cancer, and angina. Fibromyalgia was last on the list of 38. So, you may be right if you think your doctor does not understand that fibromyalgia is important. As a person who has the disease, you are an important resource in helping to educate your doctor about the significant impact that fibromyalgia can have. If she is not comfortable managing your fibromyalgia, look for someone who is (see the resources in Chapter 13).

BE AN EFFECTIVE COMMUNICATOR

You probably can't make your visit last longer, but you *can* use your time effectively. Become an effective communicator to help inform and educate your doctor about the importance of fibromyalgia and your symptoms. Become your own best advocate: Make sure that your concerns are heard, your needs are being addressed, and you understand the recommended treatments.

In most cases, your doctor will be a good resource for managing your fibromyalgia. In some cases, you may need to ask for a referral to a specialist. Most doctors are open to getting a second opinion. Seeing another physician is not a sign of failure for you or your doctor. If he suggests that you should see someone else, you shouldn't feel abandoned or think he won't treat your other health problems. Fibromyalgia can be frustrating for patients *and* their doctors. Sometimes your doctor may seem disinterested when, in fact, he has run out of ideas. This is a great time for a fresh look. The communication techniques described in this chapter can be helpful for sharing information with your doctor and talking about where to turn when you hit a stumbling block.

Is Poor Communication an Issue Between You and Your Doctor?

At your appointments, do find yourself thinking:

1. My doctor just doesn't get it when I try to tell him about my fibro symptoms.

2. He has no idea how my life is affected by fibromyalgia.

3. I never get to ask the questions that are really important to me.

4. His directions are always vague and unclear.

5. Talking to my doctor is like talking to a wall.

6. He has the bedside manner of a rock.

If you typically find yourself leaving your doctor's office feeling frustrated and having these kinds of thoughts, you need to develop a better way to communicate.

Develop Good Communication Skills

The 18th century theologian, philosopher, and scientist Joseph Priestley is credited with having said, "The more elaborate our means of communication, the less we communicate." In today's age of smartphones, teleconferencing, electronic media, and the Internet, this statement seems quite modern. Despite all the communication tools available, we still have trouble during conversations with our health care providers.

The good news is that you *can* improve communications with your health care provider—even if she is a poor communicator. By using effective communication strategies yourself, you can vastly improve the exchange of information during your typical doctor visits. Plus, when you use effective communication strategies, it actually teaches your health care provider how to communicate more effectively with you and her other patients.

Make a Written List

It's easy to get sidetracked or feel rushed during appointments and forget to share important information or ask key questions. Lists are ter-

Tips for Successful Communication

You have limited face-to-face time with your doctor—so make that time count by focusing on key concerns:

▶ Ask questions that are the most concerning to you right now.

▶ Save less urgent questions for later visits.

▶ Use direct and specific questions.

▶ Open up about what's bothering you.

▶ Restate what you hear your doctor saying to make sure you understand.

▶ Keep your doctor informed about your fibromyalgia, your other health issues, and the impact that fibromyalgia has on your daily life and long-term plans.

rific memory aids. As you prepare for a doctor visit, make a list of the information you want to share—your most troublesome symptoms, any medications and other treatments you have tried and those you're still using, and any other key concerns. Be sure to include non-prescription medications and supplements in your list of medications, and note the dose for each. Also, include a list of questions that need to be answered and concerns you want addressed.

Prioritize Your Symptoms—Be Prepared

Franklin Delano Roosevelt perhaps said it best: "Be sincere; be brief; be seated." When you have a complicated problem such as fibromyalgia, with lots of bothersome symptoms, you would need several hours to completely address all of your concerns. Unfortunately, you'll probably only have the usual 20 minutes, so use this time wisely and get your most important questions answered first.

Limit yourself to bringing only a few important questions to your appointment. A good target is to focus on three pressing concerns.

If you really want complete and thoughtful answers from your doctors, start your conversations with this statement: "There are three things I'd like to talk to you about today."

Don't expect to get everything addressed during one visit. Before your visit, decide what your three most pressing concerns are, and limit yourself to asking questions about them. Once your doctor knows that you only want to discuss three issues, you'll probably get more informative answers. Save less pressing questions for a later visit.

Ask Direct Questions and Say What You Mean

If you want to get a clear answer, ask a direct question. When men listen to women talking, they often conclude that women spend a lot of time talking *around* issues, hoping to gently lead listeners to a question, rather than just blurting it out. Men often ask, "Why can't women just say what they mean?" (Or, as Henry Higgins says in *My Fair Lady*, "Why can't a woman be more like a man?") When dealing with your health care provider—male or female—this is often good advice.

Use direct, specific questions to get the best responses from your doctor.

Doctors have a much easier time answering pointed questions. For example, if you're wondering why your doctor prescribed an antidepressant for your fibromyalgia after you just told him your mood was fine, don't vaguely ask, "Do you really think this will help?" He's bound to say, "Yes. See you in 3 weeks!" before bounding out the door and leaving you still baffled. Be direct and say, "I don't understand why you're suggesting an antidepressant. I don't feel depressed. Do you think I have a mental disorder?" Your doctor might look startled, but then he will probably explain which symptoms he's hoping will improve with the medication.

Speak Up and Share What's Really Bothering You

Doctors aren't mind readers; they don't know what your concerns are if you don't tell them. If you answer "no" when your doctor asks if you

Tell your health care provider what's bothering you the most. There are no silly questions. If something is causing you to worry, wonder, or lose sleep, it's important.

Getting the Answers You Need Using Direct Questions

Review the dialogues below between a woman with fibromyalgia and her doctor, and note when the woman uses vague, general questions or pointed, direct ones. Although the doctor answers both, the responses to general questions might unintentionally make the patient more worried and even annoyed that he doesn't seem to be taking her seriously. On the other hand, the doctor's answers to pointed questions help reduce the patient's concerns.

The patient's concern: My sister has some of the same symptoms; does she have fibromyalgia, too?

Using a general approach:

Patient: "Is fibromyalgia contagious?"

Doctor: "No."

Patient's interpretation: "Please don't ask me about your family."

Using a direct approach:

Patient: "My sister thinks she might have fibromyalgia, too. Did she catch it from me or does it run in families?"

Doctor: "Fibromyalgia is more common in people from the same family. There may be an inherited gene that causes fibromyalgia. Fibromyalgia is not spread like an infection, so people around you shouldn't worry about 'catching it' from you."

The patient's concern: I read that fibromyalgia causes pain, poor sleep, and fatigue, but what about my other problems?

Using a general approach:

Patient: "Do I need to have tests to check my bowels, bladder, and nerves?"

Doctor: "No."

Patient's interpretation: "The symptoms you're having aren't really important."

Using a direct approach:

Patient: "I know fibromyalgia causes pain and fatigue, but I also have problems with irritable bowel, painful urination, and patchy numbness. Are these symptoms part of my fibromyalgia or could they be something else?"

Doctor: "These symptoms are all typical of fibromyalgia. I see your other doctors already did a number of tests to make sure they weren't caused by another condition. Today, let's focus on your sleep, and at the next visit we'll start looking into something for your bowel problems."

The patient's concern: Why did my doctor prescribe an antidepressant for fibromyalgia when I don't have a mood problem?

Using a general approach:

Patient: "Do you think a mood pill will help my fibromyalgia?"

Doctor: "Oh, yes. This is the best treatment for problems like yours."

Patient's interpretation: "You obviously just have emotional problems!"

Using a direct approach:

Patient: "Why did you give me a mood elevator when my mood is fine?"

Doctor: "Antidepressants correct imbalances in brain chemicals that are important for mood and also for pain and sleep. Even when your mood is not a major problem, antidepressants are often helpful for fibromyalgia symptoms. I don't expect this to affect your mood, but I want you to tell me if there's a change in your sleep and pain severity."

The patient's concern: Why are you asking me to see a psychologist? Do you think I'm making up my symptoms?

Using a general approach:

Patient: "You want me to see a psychologist?"

Doctor: "Psychologists are helpful for people with problems like yours."

Patient's interpretation: "You're a nut and you need a shrink."

Using a direct approach:

Patient: "Why do I need to see a psychologist? Do you think I have emotional problems?"

Doctor: "I don't think you have a psychiatric problem. In addition to helping people who might have mood or other similar issues, psychologists have also been trained to teach important pain management skills that help change the way the brain and mind respond to pain. These techniques, such as cognitive behavioral therapy, relaxation techniques, and stress management are helpful in reducing fibromyalgia symptoms."

(continued on next page)

The patient's concern: Will I lose the ability to walk, or need to use a wheelchair?

Using a general approach:

Patient: "Should I expect things to get worse?"

Doctor: "Fibromyalgia is nothing to worry about."

Patient's interpretation: "Is he not taking me seriously, or is the prognosis so bad he won't tell me?"

Using a direct approach:

Patient: "Will fibromyalgia cause me to lose the use of my arms or legs? Will I still be able to take care of my family and myself?"

Doctor: "Fibromyalgia doesn't lead to loss of brain function, strength, your ability to walk, or anything else. We may need to adjust the way you do some things at work or around the house so the pain and fatigue don't hold you back from doing what you need and want to do."

have any unanswered questions or concerns, he really believes that you don't have any outstanding issues.

If you doctor asks about your concerns, open up and share them. If he *doesn't* ask, bring up issues yourself. You can say things like, "Before you leave, doctor, I'm really worried about . . . ."

If you're especially worried about something, be sure to ask. For example:

▶ "Do you think my symptoms could be caused by cancer?"
▶ "My sister thinks no one can possibly have as many problems as I do and that I'm probably just making them up. What do you think?"
▶ "Will I still be able to work with fibromyalgia?"
▶ "How can I keep up with everything I need to do around the house when I'm so exhausted?"
▶ "I think that new medication you started me on is making me sick."

Be a Good Reflector—Restate What You Hear for Clarification

A good way to make sure that you understand what your health care provider tells you is to rephrase what he says in order to be certain you heard it right; for example:

▶ "You're saying the pain, fatigue, bouts of diarrhea, and feeling like I'm in a fog are all part of fibromyalgia, and not caused by something serious, such as cancer or infection, right?"

▶ "When you say to take this pill every day for fibromyalgia do you mean to take it every single day or only on those days where my symptoms are especially bad?"

Rephrase what you hear your doctor saying, in your own words, to make sure you understand.

These questions help clarify what your doctor tells you, and what you need to do to improve your health.

SHARE ALL ESSENTIAL INFORMATION AT YOUR FIRST VISIT

Make sure you tell your doctor everything about your fibromyalgia and any other health concerns. Tell your doctor about your symptoms, including:

▶ Pain severity and locations
▶ How many hours you usually sleep at night, and whether your sleep is restful
▶ Whether you have problems with fatigue
▶ Whether you have bowel or bladder symptoms
▶ How your mood has been
▶ What you consider to be your worst two fibromyalgia symptoms

▶ How fibromyalgia affects your life—what you're not doing because of fibromyalgia, what you're still doing but may not be doing as well, and where your fibromyalgia holds you back

Make sure you also tell your doctor about:

▶ Any other medical conditions you're being treated for
▶ Other health problems you're having
▶ All of the medications you take—including prescription, over-the-counter, and natural remedies, such as herbs and supplements
▶ Any other treatment you're getting
▶ Plans for pregnancy

Information to Take to Your First Visit to a New Doctor*

Name: Date:

My main concern today is:

I'm also having these other symptoms:

Treatments I've tried in the past are:

These are my other health problems:

These are my current medications
(include non-prescription drugs
and supplements):

I'm allergic to:

My gynecology information is:

What's really worrying most today is:

*You can download this document at www.diamedicapub.com

Sample Completed Information Box

Name: Mary Smith

Date: May 14, 2011

My main concern today is: I think I have fibromyalgia. I have terrible pain and can't sleep.

I'm also having these other symptoms: Problems with diarrhea and constipation. Migraines twice a week. Painful menstrual periods.

Treatments I've tried in the past are:
Tylenol®—useless
Ultram®—mildly helpful for pain
Elavil®—made me dizzy and constipated

These are my other health problems:
High blood pressure
Mildly elevated cholesterol

These are my current medications (include non-prescription drugs and supplements)
Lotensin® 10 mg once a day
Pravastatin® 40 mg once a day
Fish oil 1500 mg three times a day
Coenzyme Q10 100 mg once a day

I'm allergic to:
Latex
Cats

My gynecology information is:
Last menstrual period May 8
Using a diaphragm and condoms
Last gyn exam January 2011
Last mammogram June 2010

What's really worrying most today is: I've been getting really frustrated and snapping at my family and coworkers. I've missed four workdays this month for pain and I'm afraid I'm going to get fired.

QUESTIONS TO ASK AT EVERY VISIT—UNDERSTAND YOUR SYMPTOMS AND HOW TO TREAT THEM

When you leave each appointment, make sure you can answer all of these questions:

▶ Which of my symptoms are caused by fibromyalgia?
▶ What non-drug treatments do I need to focus on?

▶ How should I take my medication?

▶ How long should the medicine take to work?

▶ What side effects should I watch for?

▶ When is my next office visit?

Don't be afraid to say you don't understand why something was prescribed for you. If you don't understand why a treatment is prescribed, you probably won't use it carefully or consistently. Your doctor should be able to clearly explain the reason for a specific treatment.

Also, if you're interested in hearing about a specific therapy and maybe trying it, ask whether it might be appropriate for you. Most doctors are eager to consider every treatment that might help you get better, so don't feel as if you might be embarrassing her by asking about different treatments.

UNDERSTAND YOUR TREATMENT OPTIONS

Fibromyalgia treatment is often complicated. You may need to take more than one medication. You may also be prescribed non-drug treatments, changes in your sleep habits and diet, and an exercise program. Doctors often start treatments in stages—giving you one or two new things to try at each visit, rather than starting too many options at once.

Some physicians will have a nurse explain the medication instructions. Feel free to ask for written instructions. Also, ask your pharmacist to clarify any questions that weren't asked or answered in the doctor's office.

SUMMARY

▶ Communication is a two-way street, but a much more productive exchange of information and ideas occurs when at least one person uses effective communication skills.

▶ Prepare for each doctor visit. Write down your questions and select two or three that need to be answered first.

▶ Bring a list of all your medications to every visit. Also, bring your logs for any non-drug treatments you're tracking, such as exercise or relaxation training.

▶ Don't be discouraged if all of your questions are not answered right away. Trying to do too much at once can be overwhelming, both for you and your doctor.

▶ Be open about your concerns and don't be afraid to ask your doctor about new treatments you have heard about.

13

Where to Get More Information—A Guide to Fibromyalgia Resources

Knowledge is power. The more you know about fibromyalgia and how to take care of yourself, the more you will get relief from your symptoms.

Fibromyalgia expert Dr. Carol Burckhardt found that patients who received education about fibromyalgia and effective self-management techniques—such as exercises, relaxation, and stress management—showed significant short- and long-term improvements in fibromyalgia scores. In her study, approximately three of four people who received education found that it had a positive impact on their fibromyalgia, including significant improvements in physical functioning and the number of days during which they felt well. Almost all were successfully exercising for at least 20 minutes, 3 days per week, and most were using relaxation techniques. This study helped to show that learning more about fibromyalgia produces real, tangible results.

Your health care provider can be an excellent resource, and you can find additional information through a wide range of Internet and print resources. This information can help you talk with your doctor when your treatment program needs to change. Be sure to talk to your health care provider about information from other sources, so that you are in agreement about your treatment options.

INTERNET RESOURCES

Reliable Internet resources are a great way to gather information and connect you with others who share your symptoms.

PatientsLikeMe

http://www.patientslikeme.com
This interesting website helps link people with life-changing illnesses, including people with fibromyalgia. The researchers who developed this website conducted a study to determine whether patients found the site beneficial, and published their findings in the *Journal of Medical Internet Research*. Surveys were completed by 150 people with fibromyalgia; 147 of them were women. The people who visited PatientsLikeMe found the site worthwhile:

- ▶ They learned what side effects to expect from treatments.
- ▶ They were able to connect with someone else who had used a therapy they were considering, and they received good information about what to expect with a new treatment.
- ▶ Some people also appreciated the patient profile they could print out, detailing their symptoms, to use as a communication tool with their health care providers.

Internet resources are not a replacement for getting information from your doctor. Hopefully, resources such as PatientsLikeMe can help you better determine what concerns need to be addressed and provide a springboard for helpful conversations about your unique health issues.

Although the Internet offers a lot of helpful information on fibromyalgia, you can also find inaccurate and unreliable information online. Websites managed by nationally recognized organizations and reputable medical centers, such as the Mayo Clinic and Johns Hopkins, generally provide good information.

Beware of websites that sell fibromyalgia therapies. Sites claiming to have "fibromyalgia cures" or that sell treatments offering improvements that sound too good to be true are usually unreliable and should probably be avoided. If you have fibromyalgia, you already know that treating fibromyalgia is hard work, and there is no "quick fix."

Reliable Websites

Fibromyalgia Information and Practical Advice

▶ National Fibromyalgia Association
http://www.fmaware.org
▶ National Fibromyalgia Partnership, Inc.
http://fmpartnership.org
▶ Health Central's Chronic Pain Connection
http://www.chronicpainconnection.com
Offers a fibromyalgia-specific portal
http://www.healthcentral.com/chronic-pain/fibromyalgia.html
▶ The American Academy of Family Physicians patient resource site
http://familydoctor.org
▶ Johns Hopkins Arthritis Center
http://www.hopkins-arthritis.org
▶ About.com has information on fibromyalgia and chronic fatigue
http://chronicfatigue.about.com.

Exercise

▶ Exercise DVDs you can order and a helpful, free, downloadable exercise guide on exercising with chronic pain are available through the DVD tab at the Fibromyalgia Information Foundation's website at http://myalgia.com.
▶ http://www.fibromyalgiaexercise.net/
▶ Articles and research studies on exercise in fibromyalgia are linked at The FMS Community webpage at http://www.fmscommunity.org/ex.htm.

▶ Get free educational pamphlets for exercise recommendations during pregnancy at the American Congress of Obstetricians and Gynecologists website by typing in the search word "exercise" and looking for the ACOG Education Pamphlets. The website is found at http://www.acog.org/.

Relaxation Exercises

▶ You can listen to licensed psychologist Dr. Buse walk you through relaxation exercises by visiting the website http://www.maxalt.com, clicking on the "Help You Can Use" link, and then clicking on the "Relaxation Podcasts" link. (Maxalt® is a triptan drug used to treat migraines. Migraines can also be treated effectively with relaxation techniques.)

Sleep Advice

▶ National Sleep Foundation at http://www.sleepfoundation.org
▶ Sleep hygiene tips are provided under the disease category of fibromyalgia at the National Pain Foundation website at http://www.nationalpainfoundation.org.
▶ Fibromyalgia-specific sleep advice can be found by searching for "sleep" at the National Fibromyalgia Association website at http://www.fmaware.org.

BMI Calculators

▶ http://www.nhlbisupport.com/bmi/
▶ http://www.bmi-calculator.net/
▶ http://www.bmicalculator.org/

Monitor Your Progress

▶ The American Chronic Pain Association provides a fibromyalgia symptom log with both an online tracking tool and printable version. This tool monitors pain, fatigue, stiffness, mood, activities, and more. Available at http://www.theacpa.org by entering the term "Fibrolog" into the "Resource Finder" search box.

Tips on Preparing for Elective Surgery

▶ Any surgery puts significant stress on your body. When you have fibromyalgia, even what your doctor may consider to be "minor surgery" can result in unpleasant pain flares. The Fibromyalgia Information Foundation provides practical tips for preparing for surgery to help reduce fibro flares after surgery and treat flares that do occur at http://www.myalgia.com/surgery_guidance.htm.

BOOKS

Fibromyalgia Information and Practical Advice

▶ *Women Living with Fibromyalgia*, by fibromyalgia sufferer Mari Skelly

▶ *Fibromyalgia for Dummies*, by rheumatologist Roland Staud, MD, and writer Christine Adamec

▶ *What Your Doctor May Not Tell You About Fibromyalgia*, by endocrinologist R. Paul St. Amand, MD and medical assistant Claudia Craig Marek

▶ *The Cleveland Clinic Guide to Fibromyalgia*, by rheumatologist William Wilke, MD

▶ *The Complete Idiot's Guide to Fibromyalgia, 2nd edition*, by co-founder of the National Fibromyalgia Association Lynne Matallana, PhD, and psychologist Laurence Bradley, PhD

Exercise

▶ *Exercises for Fibromyalgia: The Complete Exercise Guide for Managing and Lessening Fibromyalgia Symptoms*, by fitness expert William Smith

▶ *Yoga for Fibromyalgia: Move, Breath, and Relax to Improve Your Quality of Life*, by yoga instructor Shoosh Lettick Crotzer

- *Yoga for Pain Relief: Simple Practices to Calm Your Mind & Heal Your Chronic Pain*, by yoga instructor and psychologist Kelly McGonigal, PhD
- *Fibromyalgia: Simple Relief Through Movement*, by counselor and psychophysiologist Stacie Bigelow, MA
- *Water Exercises for Fibromyalgia*, by fitness instructor Ann Rosenstein

Diet

- *Foods That Help Win the Battle Against Fibromyalgia: Ease Everyday Pain and Fight Fatigue*, by naturopath and nutritionist Deirdre Rawlings, PhD
- *The Fibromyalgia Cookbook*, by fibromyalgia sufferer Sheeley Ann Smith

Sleep

- *Say Goodnight to Insomnia*, by sleep specialist Gregg Jacobs, PhD

Fatigue

- *From Fatigued to Fantastic, 3rd edition*, by internist Jacob Teitelbaum, MD
- *The Harvard Medical School Guide to a Good Night's Sleep*, by sleep specialist Lawrence Epstein, MD

Relaxation and Stress Management

- *The Mindfulness Solution to Pain*, by psychologist Jackie Gardner-Nix
- *The Relaxation & Stress Reduction Workbook*, by psychologist Martha Davis
- *Managing Pain Before It Manages You* by Margaret A. Caudill, MD

▶ *Full Catastrophe Living: Using the Wisdom of Your Body and Mind to Face Stress, Pain, and Illness* by Jon Kabat-Zinn, PhD

▶ *Mindfulness for Beginners*, an audio CD by psychologist Jon Kabat-Zinn

Pregnancy and Nursing

▶ *Fibromyalgia and Female Sexuality*, by fibromyalgia sufferer Marline Emmal

▶ *Breastfeeding: Lifesaving Techniques and Advice for Every Stage of Nursing*, by educator Suzanne Fredregill

▶ *Drugs in Pregnancy and Lactation: A Reference Guide to Fetal and Neonatal Risk, 8th edition*, by obstetrician Gerald Griggs, MD and colleagues

▶ *Medications and Mothers' Milk: a Manual of Lactational Pharmacology, 14th edition*, by pharmacist Thomas Hale, PhD

▶ *The ABCs of Breastfeeding: Everything a Mom Needs to Know for a Happy Nursing Experience*, by nurse Stacey Rubin, MN

Herbal Therapies

▶ *Alternative Treatments for Fibromyalgia & Chronic Fatigue Syndrome, 2nd edition*, by fibromyalgia sufferer Mari Skelly and Helen Walker

▶ *Clinical Botanical Medicine: Revised & Expanded*, by naturopath Eric Yarnell and colleagues

▶ *The ABC Clinical Guide to Herbs*, edited by founder of the American Botanical Council Mark Blumenthal

▶ *Herbal Medicines in Pregnancy and Lactation: An Evidence-based Approach*, by Edward Mills and colleagues

▶ *The Nursing Mother's Herbal*, by nurse and botanist Sheila Humphrey, RN

Support Groups

Research proves that participating in support groups—including online groups—empowers people. A recent analysis of what people liked and disliked about online support groups found more benefits than complaints.

How active do you need to be if you join a support group? A study by Dr. van Uden-Kraan and colleagues compared benefits from online support groups between those who were active group participants and posted information, and those who just read the information without contributing. They called this latter group "lurkers." As you'd expect, the active group members received great benefit from the site, but so did the lurkers. Both groups felt they learned good information, were better informed and more confident in their relationship with their health care providers, felt more optimistic about being able to control symptoms, and developed improved self-esteem. The active posters, however,

---

What Do People with Fibromyalgia Think About Online Support Groups?

What People Like About Support Groups

Support groups are a great way to exchange information.

People get emotional support.

People find a sense of recognition. and understanding from others who also have fibromyalgia.

People appreciate sharing their experiences with others.

People feel like they're helping others in the group.

What People Dislike About Support Groups

People worry about whether the information they hear is reliable.

People don't like hearing about more negative aspects of fibromyalgia, such as others becoming more disabled.

People are irritated by group participants who are chronic complainers.

were generally more satisfied with the support group and developed a better sense of finding recognition for their symptoms, exchanging information, and feeling improved social well-being. The "take home" messages were:

▶ You can benefit from being part of an online support group, even if you're reluctant or shy about posting information.
▶ You'll probably find the support group more helpful if you participate actively.

Finding a Support Group Near You

The National Fibromyalgia Association website at http://www.fmaware .org has links on its homepage where you can click to find local support groups and information on starting a support group.

Online Support

▶ WebMD Fibromyalgia Community
http://exchanges.webmd.com/fibromyalgia-exchange
▶ Daily strength support group
http://www.dailystrength.org/c/Fibromyalgia/support-group
▶ MDJunction
http://www.mdjunction.com/fibromyalgia

FINDING FIBROMYALGIA PROVIDERS

Health care providers interested in treating fibromyalgia can be found at these websites:

▶ National Fibromyalgia Association website
http://www.fmaware.org

▶ Fibromyalgia Information Foundation's website
http://myalgia.com

FINDING A THERAPIST

▶ American Psychological Association
http://www.apa.org/
▶ Association for Behavioral and Cognitive Therapies
http://www.abct.org/Home/
▶ American Headache Society Resources page
http://www.achenet.org/
▶ The Association for Behavioral and Cognitive Therapies website
has a link to find a behavioral therapist near you. Here's its website
link: http://www.abct.org/Home/.

References

Chapter 1

Frequency of Fibromyalgia

Senna ER, De Barros AL, Silva EO, et al. Prevalence of rheumatic diseases in Brazil: A study using the COPCORD approach. *J Rheumatol* 2004;31:594–7.

Lawrence RC, Fleson DT, Helmick CG, et al. Estimates of the prevalence of arthritis and other rheumatic conditions in the United States. Part II. *Arthritis Rheumat* 2008;58:26–35.

McNally JD, Matheson DA, Bakowsky VS. The epidemiology of self-reported fibromyalgia in Canada. *Chronic Dis Can* 2006;27:9–16.

Branco JC, Bannwarth B, Failde I, et al. Prevalence of fibromyalgia: A survey of five European countries. *Semin Arthritis Rheumat* 2010;39:448–53.

Symptoms Commonly Occurring in People with Fibromyalgia

Van Ittersum MW, van Wilgen CP, Hilberdink WA, Groothoff JW, van der Schans CP. Illness perceptions in patients with fibromyalgia. *Patient Educ Couns* 2009;74:53–60.

London Fibromyalgia Epidemiology Study

White KP, Speechley M, Harth M, Ostbye T. Testing an instrument to screen for fibromyalgia syndrome in general population studies:

The London Fibromyalgia Epidemiology Study Screening Questionnaire. *J Rheumatol* 1999;26:880–4.

Quality of Life

Silverman S, Dukes EM, Johnston SS, et al. The economic burden of fibromyalgia: Comparative analysis with rheumatoid arthritis. *Curr Med Res Opin* 2009;25:829–40.

Effect of Unpredictable Symptoms

Alvarez RP, Chen G, Bodurka J, Kaplan R, Grillon C. Phasic and sustained fear in humans elicits distinct patterns of brain activity. *Neuroimage* 2011;55:389–400.

Rhudy JL, Williams AE, McCabe KM, Rambo PL, Russell JL. Emotional modulation of spinal nociception and pain: The impact of predictable noxious stimulation. *Pain* 2006;126:221–33.

Bondi CO, Rodriguez G, Gould GG, Frazer A, Morilak DA. Chronic unpredictable stress induces a cognitive deficit and anxiety-like behavior in rats that is prevented by chronic antidepressant drug treatment. *Neuropsychopharmacology* 2008;33:320–31.

CHAPTER 2

Menopause and Fibromyalgia

Waxman J, Katzkis SM. Fibromyalgia and menopause. Examination of the relationship. *Postgrad Med* 1986;80:165–71.

Gender Bias for Not Diagnosing Fibromyalgia in Men

Katz JD, Mamyrova G, Guzhva O, Furmark L. Gender bias in diagnosing fibromyalgia. *Gend Med* 2010;7:19–27.

Gender Effects on Treatment Response

Garcia-Campayo J, Magdalena J, Magallón R, et al. A meta-analysis of the efficacy of fibromyalgia treatment according to level of care. *Arthritis Res Ther* 2008;10:R81.

Arnold LM, Lu Y, Crofford LJ, et al. A double-blind, multicenter trial comparing duloxetine with placebo in the treatment of fibromyalgia patients with or without major depressive disorder. *Arthritis Rheumat* 2004;50:2974–84.

Fibromyalgia Effects on Everyday Life

Jones J, Rutledge DN, Jones KD, Matallana L, Rooks DS. Self-assessed physical function levels of women with fibromyalgia: A national survey. *Women's Health Issues* 2008;18:406–12.

Impact of Fibromyalgia on Family Members

Dogan SK, Aytur YK, Atbasoglu C. Assessment of the relatives or spouses cohabiting with the fibromyalgia patients: Is there a link regarding fibromyalgia symptoms, quality of life, general health and psychologic status? *Rheumatol Int* 2011;31:1137–42.

Steiner JL, Bigatti SM, Hernandez AM, Lydon-Lam JR, Johnston EL. Social support mediates the relations between role strains and marital satisfaction in husbands of patients with fibromyalgia syndrome. *Fam Syst Health* 2010;28:209–23.

Impact of Fibromyalgia on Employment

Al-Allaf. Work disability and health system utilization in patients with fibromyalgia syndrome. *J Clin Rheumatol* 2007;13:199–201.

Trauma and Fibromyalgia

Al-Allaf AW, Dunbar KL, Hallum NS, et al. A case-control study examining the role of physical trauma in the onset of fibromyalgia syndrome. *Rheumatology* 2002;41:450–3.

Turk DC, Okifuji A, Starz TW, Sinclair JD. Effects of type of symptom onset on psychological distress in fibromyalgia syndrome patients. *Pain* 1996;68:423–30.

Family Patterns of Fibromyalgia

Arnold LM, Hudson JI, Hess EV, et al. Family study of fibromyalgia. *Arthritis Rheum* 2004;50:944–52.

Expectations from Fibromyalgia

Van Ittersum MW, van Wilgen CP, Hilberdink WA, Groothoff JW, van der Schans CP. Illness perceptions in patients with fibromyalgia. *Patient Educ Couns* 2009;74:53–60.

Reisine S, Fifield J, Walsh, Forrest DD. Employment and health status changes among women with fibromyalgia: A five-year study. *Arthritis Care Res* 2008;59:1735–41.

CHAPTER 3

Common Symptoms with Fibromyalgia

Bennett RM, Jones J, Turk DC, Russell IJ, Matallana L. An internet survey of 2,596 people with fibromyalgia. *BMC Musculoskelet Dis* 2007;8:27.

Poor Sleep and Fibromyalgia

Roehrs T, Hyde M, Blaisdell B, Greenwald M, Roth T. Sleep loss and REM sleep loss are hyperalgesic. *Sleep* 2006;29:145–51.

Zoppi M, Maresca M. Symptoms accompanying fibromyalgia. *Reumatismo* 2008;60:217–20.

Cappelleri JC, Bushmakin AG, McDermott AM, et al. Measurement properties of the Medical Outcomes Study Sleep Scale in patients with fibromyalgia. *Sleep Med* 2009;10:766–70.

Pain, Poor Sleep, and Fatigue

Humphrey L, Arbuckel R, Mease P, et al. Fatigue in fibromyalgia: A conceptual model informed by patient interviews. *BMC Musculoskelet Disord* 2010;11:216.

Stuifbergen AK, Phillips L, Carter P, Morrison J, Todd A. Subjective and objective sleep difficulties in women with fibromyalgia syndrome. *J Am Acad Nurse Pract* 2010;22:548–56.

Postexertional Malaise and Chronic Fatigue Syndrome

Jason LA, Porter N, Hunnell J, et al. A natural history study of chronic fatigue syndrome. *Rehabil Psychol* 2011;56:32–42.

Nijs J, Almond F, De Becker P, Truijen S, Paul L. Can exercise limits prevent post-exertional malaise in chronic fatigue syndrome? An uncontrolled clinical trial. *Clin Rehabil* 2008;22:426–35.

Aaron LA, Burke MM, Buchwald D. Overlapping conditions among patients with chronic fatigue syndrome, fibromyalgia, and temporomandibular disorder. *Arch Intern Med* 2000;160:221–7.

Kishi A, Natelsom BH, Togo F, et al. Sleep stage transitions in chronic fatigue syndrome patients with or without fibromyalgia. *Conf Proc IEEE Eng Med Biol Soc* 2010:2010;5391–4.

Fibro Fog

Katz RS, Heard AR, Mills M, Leavitt F. The prevalence and clinical impact of reported cognitive difficulties (fibrofog) in patients with rheumatic disease with and without fibromyalgia. *J Clin Rheumatol* 2004;10:53–8.

Glass JM, Park DC, Minear M, Crofford LJ. Memory beliefs and function in fibromyalgia patients. *J Psychosom Res* 2005;58:263–9.

Irritable Bowel Syndrome

Hungin AS, Whorwell PJ, Tack J, Mearin F. The prevalence, patterns and impact of irritable bowel syndrome: An international survey of 40,000 subjects. *Aliment Pharmacol Ther* 2003;17:643–50.

Bladder and Sexual Symptoms

Nickel JC, Tripp DA, Pontari M, et al. Interstitial cystitis/painful bladder syndrome and associated medical conditions with an emphasis on irritable bowel syndrome, fibromyalgia and chronic fatigue syndrome. *J Urol* 2010;184:1358–63.

Orellana C, Gratacós J, Galisteo C, Larrosa M. Sexual dysfunction in patients with fibromyalgia. *Curr Rheumatol Rep* 2009;11:437–42.

Kalichman L. Association between fibromyalgia and sexual dysfunction in women. *Clin Rheumatol* 2009;28:365–9.

Identifying Symptoms Needing to Be Improved

Bennett RM, Russell J, Cappelleri JC, et al. Identification of symptom and functional domains that fibromyalgia patients would like to see improved: A cluster analysis. *BMC Musculoskelet Disord* 2010;11:134.

CHAPTER 4

Diagnosing Fibromyalgia

Wolfe F, Smythe HA, Yunus MB, et al. 1990 The American College of Rheumatology 1990 criteria for the classification of fibromyalgia. *Arthritis Rheumat* 33:160–72.

Wolfe F, Clauw DJ, Fitzcharles M, et al. Fibromyalgia criteria and severity scales for clinical and epidemiological studies: a modification of the ACR preliminary diagnostic criteria for fibromyalgia. *J Rheumatol* 2011;38:1113–22.

Häuser W, Hayo S, Biewer W, et al. Diagnosis of fibromyalgia syndrome: A comparison of Association of the Medical Scientific Societies in Germany, survey, and American College of Rheumatology criteria. *Clin J Pain* 2010;26:505–11.

Choy E, Perrot S, Leon T, et al. A patient survey of the impact of fibromyalgia and the journey to diagnosis. *BMC Health Serv Res* 2010;10:102.

Chapter 5

Nerve Changes in Fibromyalgia

Desmeules JA, Cedraschi C, Rapiti E, et al. Neurophysiologic evidence for a central sensitization in patients with fibromyalgia. *Arthritis Rheumat* 2003;48:1420–9.

Staud R, Vierck CJ, Cannon RL, Mauderli AP, Price DD. Abnormal sensitization and temporal summation of second pain (wind-up) in patients with fibromyalgia syndrome. *Pain* 2001;91:165–75.

Gracely RH, Petzke F, Wolf JM, Clauw DJ. Functional magnetic resonance imaging evidence of augmented pain processing in fibromyalgia. *Arthritis Rheumat* 2002;46:1333–43.

Muscle Changes in Fibromyalgia

Bazzichi L, Dini M, Rossi A, et al. Muscle modifications in fibromyalgia patients revealed by surface electromyography (SEMG) analysis. *BMC Musculoskelet Disord* 2009;10:36.

Genetics and Fibromyalgia

Arnold LM, Hudson JI, Hess EV, et al. Family study of fibromyalgia. *Arthritis Rheum* 2004;50:944–52.

Lee YH, Choi SJ, Ji JD, Song GG. Candidate gene studies of fibromyalgia: A systematic review and meta-analysis. *Rheumatol Int*, in press.

Potvin S, Larouche A, Normand E, et al. DRD3 Ser9Gly polymorphism is related to thermal pain perception and modulation in chronic widespread pain patients and healthy controls. *J Pain* 2009;10:969–75.

Inflammation and Fibromyalgia

Wang H, Buchner M, Moser MT, Daniel V, Schiltenwolf M. The role of IL-8 in patients with fibromyalgia: A prospective longitudinal study of 6 months. *Clin J Pain* 2009;25:1–4.

Stress and Fibromyalgia

Ablin JN, Cohen H, Clauw DJ, et al. A tale of two cities - the effect of low intensity conflict on prevalence and characteristics of musculoskeletal pain and somatic symptoms associated with chronic stress. *Clin Exp Rheumatol* 2010;28(6 suppl 63):S15–21.

Tanriverdi F, Karaca Z, Unluhizarci K, Kelestimur F. The hypothalamo-pituitary-adrenal axis in chronic fatigue syndrome and fibromyalgia syndrome. *Stress* 2007;10:13–25.

Abuse

Walsh CA, Jamieson E, MacMillan H, Boyle M. Child abuse and chronic pain in a community survey of women. *J Interpers Violence* 2007;22:1536–54.

Sachs-Ericsson N, Blazer D, Plant EA, Arnow B. Childhood sexual and physical abuse and the 1–year prevalence of medical problems in the National Comorbidity Survey. *Health Psychol* 2005;24:32–40.

Alexander RW, Bradley LA, Alarcón GC, et al. Sexual and physical abuse in women with fibromyalgia: Association with outpatient health care utilization and pain medication usage. *Arthritis Care Res* 1998;11:102–15.

Goodwin RD, Stein MB. Association between childhood trauma and physical disorders among adults in the United States. *Psychol Med* 2004;34:509–20.

Post-traumatic Stress Disorder Screener

Prins A, Ouimette P, Kimerling R, et al. The primary care PTSD screen (PC–PTSD): Development and operating characteristics. *Primary Care Psychiatry* 2003;9:9–14.

Melatonin

Korszun Am Sackett-Lundeen L, Papadopoulos E, et al. Melatonin levels in women with fibromyalgia and chronic fatigue syndrome. *J Rheumatol* 1999;26:2675–80.

Klerman EB, Goldenberg DL, Brown EN, Maliszewski AM, Alder GK. Circadian rhythms of women with fibromyalgia. *J Clin Endocrinol Metab* 2001;86:1034–9.

Growth Hormone

Cuatrecasas G, Gonzalez MJ, Alegre C, et al. High prevalence of growth hormone deficiency in severe fibromyalgia syndromes. *J Clin Endocrinol Metab* 2010;95:4331–7.

Thyroid

Bazzichi L, Rossi A, Giuliano T, et al. Association between thyroid autoimmunity and fibromyalgic disease severity. *Clin Rheumatol* 2007;26:2115–20.

Bazzichi L, Rossi A, Zirafa C, et al. Thyroid autoimmunity may represent a predisposition for the development of fibromyalgia? *Rheumatol Int*, in press.

Estrogen

Ouyang A, Wrzos HF. Contribution of gender to pathophysiology and clinical presentation of IBS: Should management be different in women? *Am J Gastroenterol* 2006;101(12 suppl):S602–9.

Colangelo K, Haig S, Bonner A, Zelenietz C, Pope J. Self-reported flaring varies during the menstrual cycle in systemic lupus erythematosus compared with rheumatoid arthritis and fibromyalgia. *Rheumatology* (Oxford) 2011;50:703–8.

Ostensen M, Rugelsjøen A, Wigers SH. The effect of reproductive events and alterations of sex hormones on the symptoms of fibromyalgia. *Scand Rheumatol* 1997;26:355–60.

Stening KD, Eriksson O, Henriksson KG, et al. Hormonal replacement therapy does not affect self-estimated pain or experimental pain responses in post-menopausal women suffering from fibromyalgia: A double-blind, randomized, placebo-controlled trial. *Rheumatology* 2011;50:544–51.

Santen RJ, Allred DC, Ardoin SP, et al. Postmenopausal hormone therapy: an endocrine society scientific statement. *J Clin Endocrinol Metab* 2010;95(suppl 1):S1–S66.

CHAPTER 6

Exercise

Busch AJ, Barber KA, Overend TJ, Peloso PM, Schachter CL. Exercise for treating fibromyalgia syndrome. *Cochrane Database Syst Rev* 2007;4:CD003786.

Etnier JL, Karper WB, Gapin JI, et al. Exercise, fibromyalgia, and fibrofog: A pilot study. *J Phys Act Health* 2009;6:239–46.

Häuser W, Klose P. Langhorst J, et al. Efficacy of different types of aerobic exercise in fibromyalgia syndrome: A systematic review and meta-analysis of randomised controlled trials. *Arthritis Res Ther* 2010;12:R79.

Altan L, Korkmaz N, Bingol U, Gunay B. Effects of Pilates training on people with fibromyalgia syndrome: A pilot study. *Arch Phys Med Rehabil* 2009;90:1983–8.

Water Therapy

Langhorst J, Musial F, Klose P, Häuser W. Efficacy of hydrotherapy in fibromyalgia syndrome—a meta-analysis of randomized controlled clinical trials. *Rheumatology* 2009;48:1155–9.

Yoga

Carson JW, Carson KM, Jones KD, et al. A pilot randomized controlled trial of the Yoga of Awareness program in the management of fibromyalgia. *Pain* 2010;15:530–9.

Hölzel BK, Carmody J, Vangel M, et al. Mindfulness practice leads to increases in regional brain gray matter density. *Psychiatry Res: Neuroimaging* 2011;191:36–43.

Tai Chi

Wang C, Schmid CH, Rones R, et al. A randomized trial of tai chi for fibromyalgia. *N Engl J Med* 2010;363:743–54.

Physical Therapy Treatments

Ekici G, Bakar Y, Akbayrak T, Yusel I. Comparison of manual lymph drainage therapy and connective tissue massage in women with fibromyalgia: A randomized controlled trial. *J Manipulative Physiol Ther* 2009;32:127–33.

Castro-Sánchez AM, Matarán-Peñarrocha GA, Granero-Molina J, et al. Benefits of massage-myofascial release therapy on pain, anxiety, quality of sleep, depression, and quality of life in patients with fibromyalgia. *Evid Based Complement Altern Med* 2011;2011: 561753.

Field T, Diego M, Cullen C, et al. Fibromyalgia pain and substance P decrease and sleep improves after massage therapy. *J Clin Rheumatol* 2002;8:72–6.

Acupuncture

Martin-Sanchez E, Torralba E, Diaz-Domínguez E, Barriga A, Martin JL. Efficacy of acupuncture for the treatment of fibromyalgia: Systematic review and meta-analysis of randomized trials. *Open Rheumatol J* 2009;3:25–9.

Ernst E, Lee MS, Choi TY. Acupuncture for insomnia? An overview of systematic reviews. *Eur J Gen Pract* 2011;17:116–23.

Huang W, Kutner N, Bliwise DL. A systematic review of the effects of acupuncture in treating insomnia. *Sleep Med Rev* 2009;13:73–104.

Chey WD, Maneerattaporn M, Saad R. Pharmacologic and complementary and alternative medicine therapies for irritable bowel syndrome. *Gut Liver* 2011;5:253–66.

CHAPTER 7

Behavioral Therapy

Thieme K, Flor H, Turk DC. Psychological pain treatment in fibromyalgia syndrome: Efficacy of operant behavioural and cognitive behavioural treatments. *Arthritis Res Ther* 2006;8:R121.

Thieme K, Turk DC, Flor H. Responder criteria for operant and cognitive-behavioral treatment of fibromyalgia syndrome. *Arthritis Rheumat* 2007;57:830–36.

Stress Management

Cornelisse S, van Stegeren AH, Joëls. Implications of psychosocial stress on memory formation in a typical male versus female student sample. *Psychoneuroendocrinology* 2011;36:569–78.

Weight Loss

Shapiro JR, Andersen DA, Danoff-Burg S. A pilot study of the effects of behavioral weight loss treatment on fibromyalgia symptoms. *J Psychosom Res* 2005;59:275–82.

Kruger J, Blanck HM, Gillespie C. Dietary and physical activity behaviors among adults successful at weight loss maintenance. *Int J Behav Nutr Phys Act* 2006;3:17.

Smoking

Weingarten TN, Podduturu VR, Hooten WM, et al. Impact of tobacco use in patients presenting to a multidisciplinary outpatient treatment program for fibromyalgia. *Clin J Pain* 2009;25:39–43.

Lee SS, Kim SH, Nah SS, et al. Smoking habits influence pain and functional and psychiatric features in fibromyalgia. *Joint Bone Spine* 2011;78:259–65.

CHAPTER 8

Mease PJ, Dundon K, Sarzi-Puttine P. Pharmacotherapy of fibromyalgia. *Best Pract Res Clin Rheumatol* 2011;25:285-97.

CHAPTER 9

Vitamins

Block SR. Vitamin D deficiency is not associated with nonspecific musculoskeletal pain syndromes including fibromyalgia. *Mayo Clin Proc* 2004;79:1585–6.

Arvold DS, Odean MJ, Dornfeld MP, et al. Correlation of symptoms with vitamin D deficiency and symptom response to cholecalciferol treatment: A randomized controlled trial. *Endrocr Pract* 2009; 15:203–12.

Bramwell B, Ferguson S, Scarlett N, Macintosh A. The use of ascorbigen in the treatment of fibromyalgia patients: A preliminary trial. *Altern Med Rev* 2000;5:455–62.

Minerals

Sendur OF, Tastaban E, Turan Y, Ulman C. The relationship between serum trace element levels and clinical parameters in patients with fibromyalgia. *Rheumatol Int* 2008;28:1117–21.

Herbs/Supplements

Fetrow CW, Avila JR. Efficacy of the dietary supplement S-adenosyl-L-methionine. *Ann Pharmacother* 2001;35:1414–25.

Sarac AJ, Gur A. Complementary and alternative medical therapies in fibromyalgia. *Curr Pharm Des* 2006;12:47–57.

Hussain SA, Al-Khalifa II, Jasim NA, Gorial FI. Adjuvant use of melatonin for treatment of fibromyalgia. *J Pineal Res* 2011;267–71.

Dotterud CK, Storrø O, Johnsen R, Oien T. Probiotics in pregnant women to prevent allergic disease: A randomized, double-blind trial. *Br J Dermatol* 2010;163:616–23.

Nakano S, Takekoshi H, Nakano M. *Chlorella* (*Chlorella pyrenoidosa*) supplementation decreases dioxin and increases immunoglobulin A concentrations in breast milk. *J Med Food* 2007;10:134–42.

Chapter 10

General Pregnancy Symptoms and Medication Use

Kelly RH, Russo J, Katon W. Somatic complaints among pregnant women cared for in obstetrics: Normal pregnancy or depressive and anxiety symptom amplification revisited? *Gen Hosp Psychiatry* 2011;23:107–13.

Glover DD, Amonkar M, Rybeck BF, Tracy TS. Prescription, over-the-counter, and herbal medicine use in a rural, obstetric population. *Am J Obstet Gyencol* 2003;188:1039–45.

Headley J, Northstone K, Simmons H, Golding J. Medication use during pregnancy: Data from the Avon Longitudinal Study of Parents and Children. *Eur J Clin Pharmacol* 2004;60:355–61.

Academy of Breastfeeding Medicine Protocol Committee. ABM clinical protocol #18: Use of antidepressants in nursing mothers. *Breastfeed Med* 2008;3:44–52.

Pregnancy and Fibromyalgia

Ostensen M, Rugelsjøen A, Wigers SH. The effect of reproductive events and alterations of sex hormone levels on the symptoms of fibromyalgia. *Scand J Rheumatol* 1997;26:355–60.

Schaefer KM. Breastfeeding in chronic illness: The voices of women with fibromyalgia. *MCN Am J Matern Child Nurs* 2004;29:248–53.

Raphael KG, Marbach JJ. Comorbid fibromyalgia accounts for reduced fecundity in women with myofascial face pain. *Clin J Pain* 2000;16:29–36.

Medications

Favrelière S. Nourrisson A, Jaafari N, Pérault Puchat MC. Treatment of depressed pregnant women by selective serotonin reuptake inhibitors: Risk for the foetus and the newborn. *Encephale* 2010;36(suppl2):D133–8.

Lund N, Pedersen LH, Henriksen TB. Selective serotonin reuptake inhibitor exposure in utero and pregnancy outcomes. *Arch Pediatr Adolesc Med* 2009;163:949–54.

Meador KJ, Baker GA, Browning N, et al. Cognitive function at 3 years of age after fetal exposure to antiepileptic drugs. *N Engl J Med* 2009;360:1597–605.

Broussard CS, Rasmussen SA, Reefhuis J, et al. Maternal treatment with opioid analgesics and risk for birth defects. *Am J Obstet Gynecol* 2011;204:314,e1–11.

Nausea Treatment

American College of Obstetricians and Gynecologists. ACOG practice bulletin #52: Nausea and vomiting of pregnancy. *Obstet Gynecol* 2004;103:803–15.

Borrelli F, Capasso R, Aviello G, Pittler MH, Izzo AA. Effectiveness and safety of ginger in the treatment of pregnancy-induced nausea and vomiting. *Obstet Gynecol* 2005;105:849–56.

Chuang C, Doyle P, Wang J, et al. Herbal medicines used during the first trimester and major congenital malformations. An analysis of data from a pregnancy cohort study. *Drug Saf* 2006;29:537–48.

Exercise

Juhl M, Kogevinas M, Andersen PK, Andersen AM, Olsen J. Is swimming during pregnancy a safe exercise? *Epidemiology* 2010;21:253–8.

Barakat R, Ruiz JR, Stirling JR, Zakynthinaki M, Lucia A. Type of delivery is not affected by light resistance and toning exercise training during pregnancy: A randomized controlled trial. *Am J Obstet Gynecol* 2009;201:509,e3.

Kalisiak B, Spitznagle T. What effect does an exercise program for healthy pregnant women have on the mother, fetus, and child? *PMR* 2009;1:261–6.

Sleep

Hedman C, Pohjasvaara T, Tolonen U, Suhonen-Malm AS, Myllylä VV: Effects of pregnancy on mothers' sleep. *Sleep Med* 2002;3:37–42.

da Silva JB, Nakamura MU, Cordeiro JA, Kulay LJ. Acupuncture for insomnia in pregnancy – a prospective, quasi-randomised, controlled study. *Acupuncture Med* 2005;23:47–51.

CHAPTER 11

Zachrisson O, Regland B, Jahreskog M, Kron M, Gottfries CG. A rating scale for fibromyalgia and chronic fatigue syndrome (the FibroFatigue scale). *J Psychosom Res* 2002;52:501–9.

Bastien CH, Vallières A, Morin CM. Validation of the Insomnia Severity Index as an outcome measure for insomnia research. *Sleep Med* 2001;2:297–307.

Parker G, Hilton T, Bains J, Hadzi-Pavlovic D. Cognitive-based measures screening for depression in the medically ill: The DMI-10 and the DMI-18. *Acta Psychiatr Scand* 2002;105:419–26.

Spitzer RL, Kroenke K, Williams JW, Löwe B. A brief measure for assessing generalized anxiety disorder. The GAD-7. *Arch Intern Med* 2006;166:1092–7.

Bennett RM, Friend R, Jones KD, et al. The Revised Fibromyalgia Impact Questionnaire (FIQR): Validation and psychometric properties. *Arthritis Res Ther* 2009;11:R120.

Bennett RM, Bushmakin AG, Cappelleri JC, Zlateva G, Sadosky AB: Minimal clinically important difference in the fibromyalgia impact questionnaire. *J Rheumatol* 2009, 36:1304–11.

Yang M, Morin CM, Schaefer K, Wallenstein GV. Interpreting score differences in the Insomnia Severity Index: Using health-related outcomes to define the minimally important difference. *Curr Med Res Opin* 2009;25:2487–94.

Index

Note: Boldface numbers indicate tables and illustrations.